"*Good food is very often,
even most often, simple food*"
Anthony Bourdain

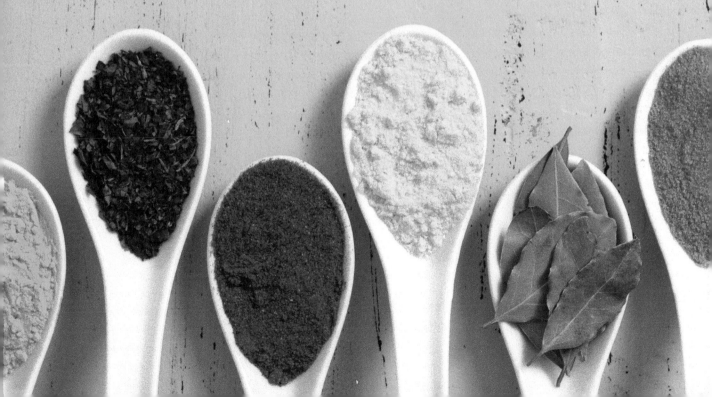

INTRODUCTION

The ketogenic diet is becoming increasingly popular, being one of the most searched for diets on Google. The idea of the diet initially seems strange to people – "eat more fat and lose more fat." People are slowly starting to realize that it is carbohydrates (particularly processed carbs) that are causing massive health problems, the main one being type 2 diabetes. By sticking to a low-carb diet, there are numerous benefits, including:

» Accelerated fat loss

» Lower cholesterol

» Lower blood sugar

» Increased levels of energy and vitality

» Improved mental focus (ketogenic diets were initially used for epilepsy)

Unfortunately, just because the diet works it does not mean people will stick to it. Particularly when it asks you to forgo habits that have been formed over many decades – "eating and cooking carbohydrates." In the fast world we live in today, people want things "quick and easy," carbohydrates provided a great way to serve this need, Cereal, bread, pasta, potatoes, chips, and so on have habitually become the "quick and easy" thing to eat and snacks like chocolate have become the emotional reward.

To help you on your ketogenic journey, I wanted to make it as quick and easy as possible, but without sacrificing any of the flavor. I want you to look forward to enjoying your keto food.

Why 6 Ingredients or Less?

I decided to write this book and develop these recipes as a way to provide easy alternatives to traditionally tedious recipes. I find that a lot of people are just too busy to prepare fancy meals each night and that most of us do not have the time to spend hours at the grocery store picking up large lists of ingredients to prep each meal. In this book, you will find that each recipe contains 6 ingredients or less making it very doable no matter what day of the week it is. Here are some of the other reasons why recipes with fewer ingredients just make sense for all of us busy people.

» **Makes Eating Keto Easier:** Less time and fewer ingredients means life made easier. Any time we can make eating keto easier, we definitely should. With fewer ingredients, eating keto is much easier as there is less of a chance for a higher carb count.

» **Food Prep:** You are more likely to do some food prep when you know you can create a meal quickly and with minimal ingredients. This will make it much easier for you to have a healthy keto-friendly meal ready and available during the busy workweek.

» **Fewer Grocery Trips:** I know some people who head to the grocery store multiple times per week because they run out of ingredients and food for the week. When you have recipes that don't require too many ingredients, you are more likely to get all of your shopping done in one trip, saving you even more time during the workweek.

I hope this book serves as useful resource for you when you need some quick and easy recipes. I know it has helped me balance my schedule better during the week while also staying on track with my keto diet.

Bonus – Keto Sweet Eats

I am delighted you have chosen my book to help you start or continue on your keto journey. Temptation by sweet treats can knock you off course so, to help you stay on the keto track, I am pleased to offer you three mini ebooks from my "Keto Sweet Eats Series," completely free of charge. These three mini ebooks cover how to make everything from keto chocolate cake to keto ice cream to keto fat bombs so you don't have to feel like you are missing out, whatever the occasion.

Simply visit the link below to get your free copy of all three mini ebooks …

http://ketojane.com/6ingred1

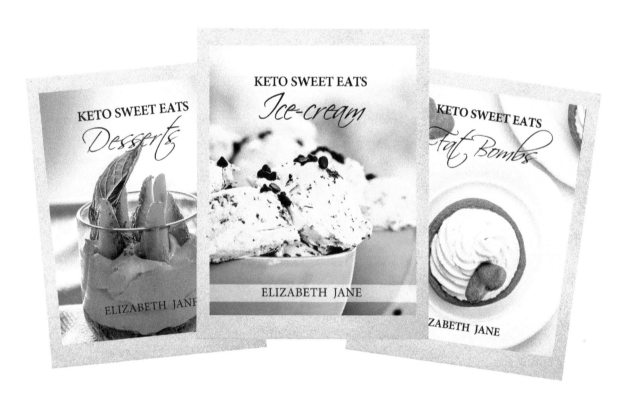

TABLE OF CONTENTS

RECIPE NOTES

Ingredients vs. Essentials

When trying to create a 6-ingredient cookbook, I looked at other examples and, unfortunately, what I saw was very bland. These were mostly basic recipes, such as scrambled eggs (eggs, milk, butter, salt, and pepper) and chicken Caesar salad (plain chicken breast, 2 types of lettuce, cheese, salt, and pepper). It was clear that it would be very difficult to make tasty food if basic ingredients like salt and black pepper were included in the 6.

Instead, I have separated "ingredients" and "essentials." Essentials are ingredients that most people would commonly have in their cupboard: salt, pepper, cooking oil, and butter. Some people may call this cheating – technically they are an ingredient – but doing this has allowed me to create much more flavorful and delicious recipes.

TAILORING THE RECIPES TO FIT YOUR PREFERENCES

These recipes have been created to be:

1. Easy to make

2. Delicious

3. Easy to find ingredients

However, there is not a one-size-fits-all recipe as everyone has different tastes, some have allergies, and not everyone will be able to get all of the ingredients. Consider the recipes as a guideline that you can then customize to your own taste or what you have in the house.

» Do not like cilantro? Consider switching it with parsley or leave it out entirely.

» Do not have any pink rock salt in the house? Just use some normal table salt instead.

» Do not like venison? Try beef instead.

» Prefer your eggs a bit runnier? Cook them for slightly less time.

» Do not want to cook 4 servings? Simply halve the ingredients and only cook 2.

» Do not have a spiralizer? Just cut into strips or use a vegetable peeler.

I have included some suggestions throughout for alternatives, but could not list every single one. Only you know what your preferences are, so have some fun with it and play around with different ingredients and recipes.

Also consider mixing up the recipes, they have been designed to be flexible. Mix some of the main dishes with a side dish and, of course, treat yourself — these are some of my favorite desserts.

Once again, thank you for downloading. I appreciate you allowing me to help you. I'd also appreciate any feedback you have. Please either leave an honest review by visiting http://ketojane.com/6review or email me at elizabeth@ketojane.com

Dietary Labels

Within this book, you will notice that there are dietary labels. These will indicate whether a recipe is gluten-free, or paleo. Although the majority of the recipes are gluten-free, always be sure to check the food label on the ingredients you buy due to the variations in certain product ingredients. If a recipe is not paleo-compliant, most recipes contain suggestions for how to make a recipe paleo-friendly. Some recipes require dairy, however, and substitutions cannot be made.

GF: Gluten-free
P: Paleo (There are also paleo substitutions for recipes that are not paleo-friendly)

YOU MAY ALSO LIKE

Please visit the below link for other books by the author

http://ketojane.com/books

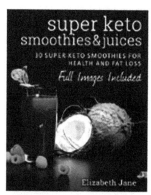
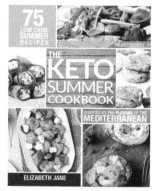
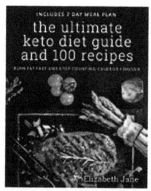

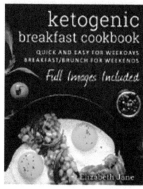
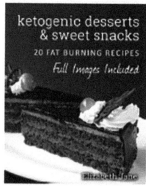
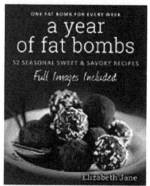

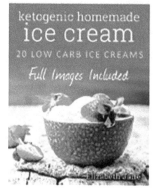
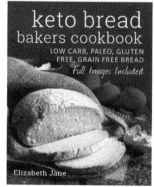
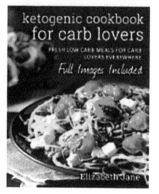

FISH / SEAFOOD

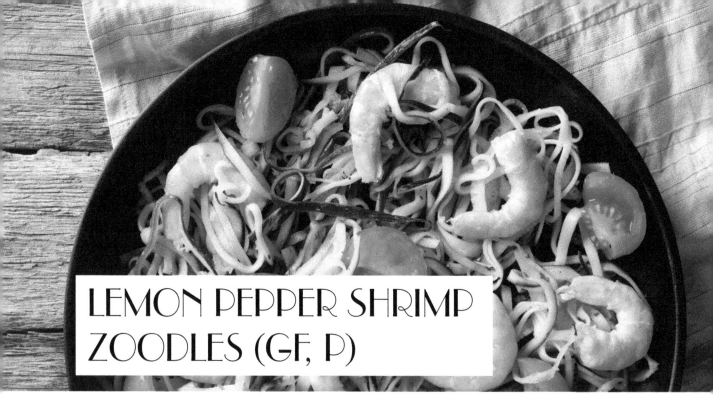

LEMON PEPPER SHRIMP ZOODLES (GF, P)

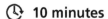 5 minutes   10 minutes   👥

INGREDIENTS

» ¾ pound large shrimp, peeled and deveined
» 1 lemon, juiced and zested
» 1 tablespoon fresh parsley, chopped
» 2 medium zucchinis, spiralized
» 5 cherry tomatoes, quartered

Essentials

» ½ teaspoon freshly ground black pepper, or as needed to taste
» ½ teaspoon salt, or as needed to taste
» 1 tablespoon of extra virgin olive oil

DIRECTIONS

1. Mix the shrimp, lemon juice and lemon zest together in a mixing bowl and season to taste with black pepper and salt. Ensure that the shrimp is evenly coated with the ingredients.
2. Add the olive oil to a large skillet or cast iron pan over a medium-high heat. Once the oil is hot, add the shrimp and most of the parsley. Stirring often, sauté the shrimp and parsley for about 5 or 6 minutes, until the shrimp is opaque and cooked through.
3. Add the zoodles (zucchini noodles) and sauté for 2-3 minutes or until al dente. Make sure not to overcook. Mix well to get the juices well distributed into the zoodles.
4. Remove the skillet from the heat and stir in half of the remaining parsley. Divide the shrimp and zoodles evenly between four plates and garnish with the remaining fresh parsley along with the quartered cherry tomatoes on top and lemon wedges on the side.

NUTRITION FACTS (PER SERVING)

Total Carbohydrates: 6g	**Dietary Fiber: 1g**	**Net Carbs: 5g**
Protein: 24g	**Total Fat: 5g**	**Calories: 169**

12

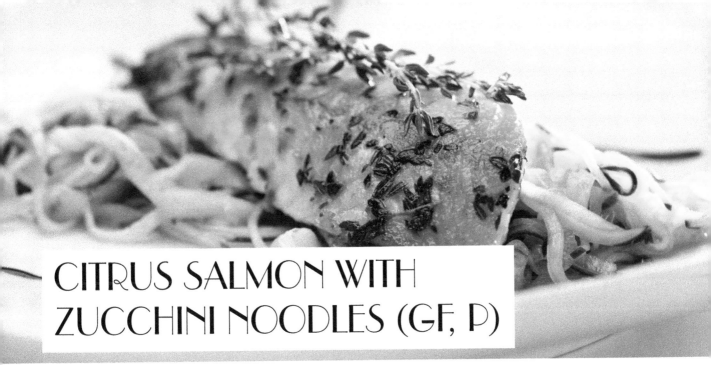

CITRUS SALMON WITH ZUCCHINI NOODLES (GF, P)

 10 minutes   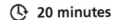 **20 minutes**

INGREDIENTS

- » 1 fresh lime, juiced and zested
- » 1 garlic clove, peeled and minced
- » 2 large salmon fillets
- » ½ teaspoon dried oregano
- » 4 medium zucchinis, spiralized

Essentials

- » Salt, to taste
- » 2 tablespoons coconut oil, for cooking

Optional / Garnish

- » Fresh thyme sprig

DIRECTIONS

1. To prepare the marinade: Heat half of the coconut oil in a pan, add the garlic clove and gradually add half the lime juice to achieve a smooth consistency. Finally, add the dried oregano.
2. Place the salmon into a glass baking dish and add the marinade. Coat each salmon fillet with the marinade and cover the dish. Transfer to the refrigerator and allow the salmon to marinate for about 3 hours.
3. Use a spiralizer, mandolin, or vegetable peeler to create noodles or strips from the zucchini.
4. Preheat the oven to 450 degrees Fahrenheit. Take the marinated salmon out of the refrigerator, ensure the salmon is skin-side down and spoon more sauce over the top of the salmon. Place the dish in the center of the oven and bake for about 11-13 minutes.
5. Sauté the zucchini in the remaining coconut oil and lime juice for about 3-4 minutes, ensuring the noodles receive a good coating of the juices.
6. Divide the zucchini noodles between two plates or bowls and pour the remaining marinade over the top. Place a salmon fillet on top of each plate or bowl of noodles. Add salt to taste and garnish with a fresh thyme sprig to serve.

NUTRITION FACTS (PER SERVING)

Total Carbohydrates: 3g	Dietary Fiber: 1g	Net Carbs: 2g
Protein: 66g	Total Fat: 41g	Calories: 656

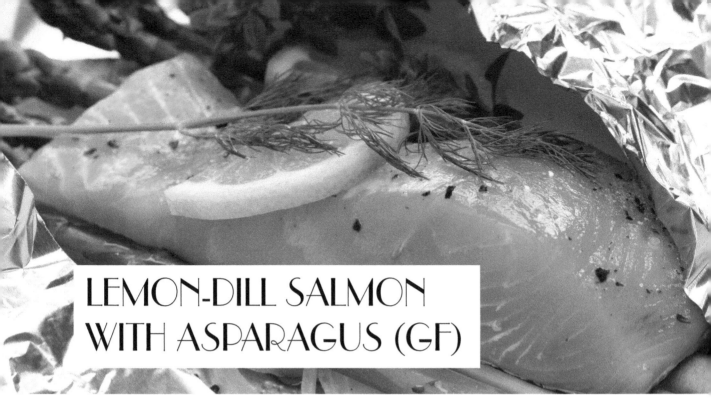

LEMON-DILL SALMON WITH ASPARAGUS (GF)

 20 minutes   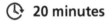 **20 minutes**

INGREDIENTS

» 2 salmon fillets
» 1 onion, peeled and sliced thin
» 12 asparagus spears, trimmed
» 2 garlic cloves, peeled and sliced
» 6 slices of lemon
» 1 teaspoon fresh dill, chopped

Essentials

» 1 tablespoon canola oil (use olive oil for a paleo version)
» Salt and coarsely ground black pepper, to taste

DIRECTIONS

1. Preheat oven to 400°F. Prepare two big sheets of aluminum foil to wrap and bake the fish.
2. Place the asparagus spears in the center of the foil. Top with the salmon fillets.
3. Season the salmon fillets with salt and pepper, add the garlic slices and drizzle with canola oil.
4. Place 2 lemon slices and the onion slices over the salmon and fold the foil over to make a packet.
5. Bake the fish in the oven for 18-20 minutes.
6. Transfer the salmon and asparagus carefully to serving plates and garnish with the remaining lemon slices and chopped dill. Enjoy!

NUTRITION FACTS (PER SERVING)

Total Carbohydrates: 13g	Dietary Fiber: 1g	Net Carbs: 11g
Protein: 35g	Total Fat: 23g	Calories: 482

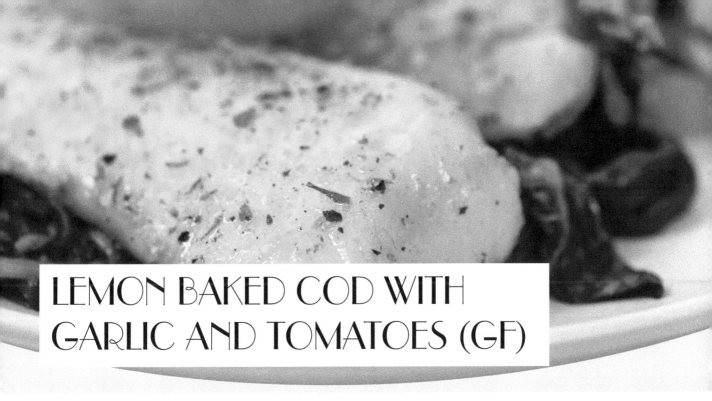

LEMON BAKED COD WITH GARLIC AND TOMATOES (GF)

 5 minutes   **15 minutes**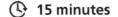

INGREDIENTS

» 2 cod fillets, about 6 ounces each (or use your favorite whitefish)
» 2 garlic cloves, peeled and minced
» 1 tablespoon fresh lemon juice
» 2 tablespoon fresh parsley, chopped
» 4 cherry tomatoes, halved
» ½ cup baby spinach leaves

Essentials

» Salt and ground black pepper, to taste
» 2 tablespoons coconut oil, for cooking
» Nonstick cooking spray (use coconut oil for a paleo version)

DIRECTIONS

1. Preheat oven to 400°F.
2. Add the coconut oil to a small pot and set over low heat.
3. When the oil begins to sizzle, add the garlic and cook for about 60 seconds.
4. Stir in the lemon juice and remove the pot from the heat.
5. Coat a glass baking dish with nonstick cooking spray.
6. Add the fish and sprinkle with salt and pepper. Rub with your hands to coat evenly.
7. Spoon the garlic mixture over the fish, sprinkle with fresh chopped parsley, add the halved tomatoes and bake for 14-16 minutes until opaque throughout.
8. Sauté the spinach in some of the juices from the fish for about 1 minute. Mix well to ensure it receives a good coating of juices.
9. Serve the fish on a bed of baby spinach and drizzle with any remaining juices.

NUTRITION FACTS (PER SERVING)

Total Carbohydrates: 7g	**Dietary Fiber: 1g**	**Net Carbs: 6g**
Protein: 19g	**Total Fat: 14g**	**Calories: 230**

15

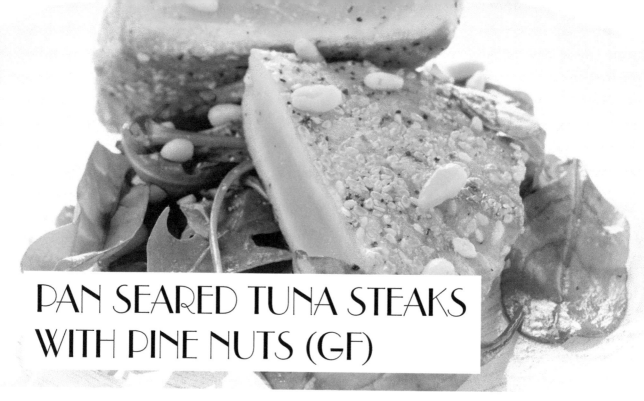

PAN SEARED TUNA STEAKS WITH PINE NUTS (GF)

 10 minutes 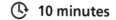 10 minutes

INGREDIENTS

» 2 fresh tuna steaks, about 3 ounces each
» 1 teaspoon chili powder
» ¼ teaspoon dried thyme
» ½ teaspoon garlic powder
» 1 tablespoon pine nuts
» Handful of arugula or your favorite greens

Essentials

» 1 tablespoon olive oil
» 1 tablespoon butter (add 1 tablespoon. more olive oil for a paleo version)
» Salt and ground black pepper, to taste

DIRECTIONS

1. Combine all of the seasonings (chili powder, dried thyme, and garlic powder) and add a dash of salt and pepper.
2. Add a little coating of olive oil to the tuna steaks and sprinkle the seasoning mixture over both sides, distributing it as evenly as possible.
3. Add the olive oil and butter to a large skillet and heat over medium-high heat.
4. Once the butter has melted and the oil is hot, add the pine nuts and the tuna steaks and cook for about 4-5 minutes on each side until blackened or cooked to your preference. The pine nuts should be soft and golden brown.
5. Serve immediately on a bed of arugula.

NUTRITION FACTS (PER SERVING)

Total Carbohydrates: 3g	Dietary Fiber: 1g	Net Carbs: 2g
Protein: 33g	Total Fat: 14g	Calories: 269

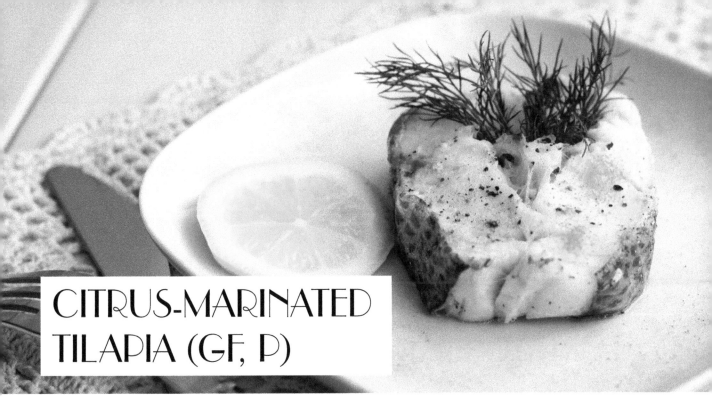

CITRUS-MARINATED TILAPIA (GF, P)

🥄 **10 minutes**   🕐 **25 minutes**   👥

INGREDIENTS

» 4 tilapia fillets, about 4 ounces each
» ¼ cup lime juice or lemon juice (do not use both)
» ¼ cup green onions, chopped
» 1 tablespoon fresh dill, chopped
» ½ teaspoon garlic powder

Essentials

» 2 tablespoons coconut oil, for cooking
» 1 tablespoon water
» Salt and coarsely ground black pepper, to taste

DIRECTIONS

1. Mix the coconut oil, green onions, lime juice or lemon juice, dill, garlic powder, and water in a baking dish. Add the fish fillets and toss with your hands to coat. Season with salt.
2. Cover with aluminum foil and let marinate in the refrigerator for at least 1 hour.
3. When ready to cook, preheat the oven to 350°F, remove the fish from the refrigerator, and bake covered in the oven for about 30 minutes until the fillets are cooked through.
4. Place the fillets on a serving plate, season with black pepper and serve. Garnish with dill, if desired.

NUTRITION FACTS (PER SERVING)

Total Carbohydrates: 5g	Dietary Fiber: 1g	Net Carbs: 4g
Protein: 47g	Total Fat: 18g	Calories: 296

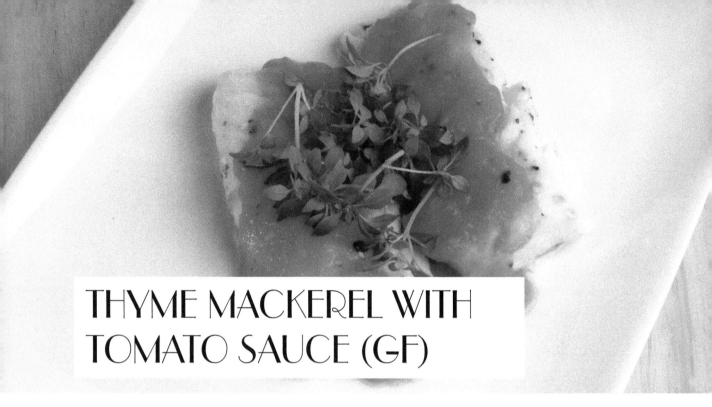

THYME MACKEREL WITH TOMATO SAUCE (GF)

 5 minutes   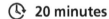 **20 minutes**

INGREDIENTS

» 2 mackerel fillets, about 4 ounces each
» 1 green onion, chopped
» 1 (14 ounce) can chopped tomatoes (use fresh tomatoes for a paleo version)
» 1 teaspoon light brown sugar (leave this out if you want or are opting for a paleo version)
» Small bunch of thyme leaves, chopped
» Fresh cilantro, for serving

Essentials

» 1 tablespoon canola oil (use olive oil for a paleo version)
» Salt and ground black pepper, to taste

DIRECTIONS

1. Add the oil to a large skillet and set over medium heat.
2. Add the onion and sauté for 4-5 minutes.
3. Add the salt, pepper, and thyme leaves, stir, and add the tomatoes.
4. When the mixture begins to boil, reduce the heat to low, and let it simmer for about 5 minutes.
5. Add the mackerel fillets to the sauce, cover, and simmer for about 10 minutes, until the fish is cooked through.
6. Top with cilantro and serve alongside sautéed or steamed vegetables.

NUTRITION FACTS (PER SERVING)

Total Carbohydrates: 7g	**Dietary Fiber: 3g**	**Net Carbs: 4g**
Protein: 22g	**Total Fat: 23g**	**Calories: 325**

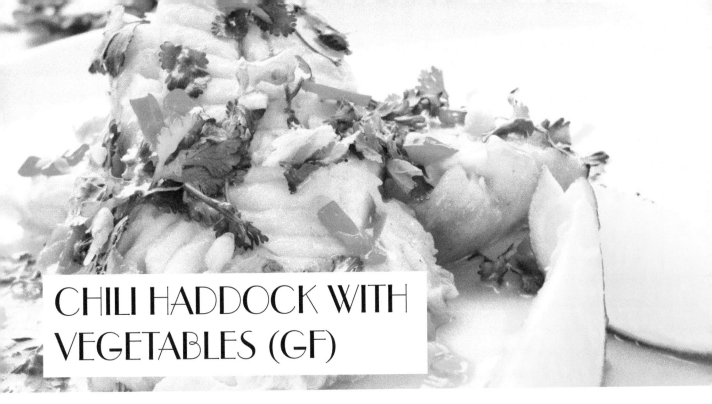

CHILI HADDOCK WITH VEGETABLES (GF)

 5 minutes   **20 minutes**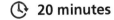

INGREDIENTS:

- » 1 teaspoon dill weed, chopped
- » 1 small onion, peeled and sliced thin
- » 2 garlic cloves, peeled and minced
- » 2 haddock fillets, about 4 ounces each (or use your favorite whitefish)
- » ½ medium red chili pepper, chopped
- » 1 cup of your favorite vegetables / greens (my favorite is arugula)

Essentials

- » 2 tablespoons olive oil
- » 1 tablespoon butter (eliminate or use more olive oil for a paleo version)
- » Salt and ground black pepper, to taste

Garnish

- » Lime wedges

DIRECTIONS:

1. In a small bowl, combine the olive oil, butter, dill, garlic, onion, chili, salt, and pepper.
2. Pour the mixture into a skillet set over medium heat.
3. When the oil begins to sizzle, add the fish and cook for 7-8 minutes per side.
4. While the fish is cooking, prepare the vegetables or greens.
5. Divide the vegetables or greens between two serving plates, top with the fish fillets, garnish with lime wedges, and enjoy.

NUTRITION FACTS (PER SERVING)

Total Carbohydrates: 9g	Dietary Fiber: 1g	Net Carbs: 8g
Protein: 33g	Total Fat: 20g	Calories: 347

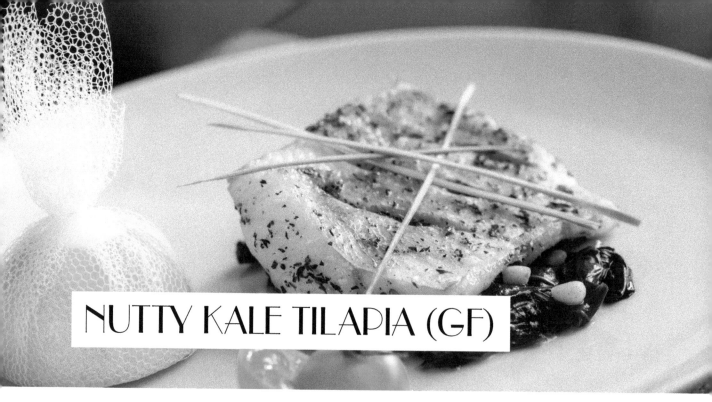

NUTTY KALE TILAPIA (GF)

 10 minutes   15-20 minutes

INGREDIENTS

» 2 tilapia fillets, about 4 ounces each
» 1 teaspoon seafood seasoning (use a compliant seasoning for a paleo version)
» ¼ cup pine nuts
» 1 bunch of kale, chopped
» ½ cup chicken broth

Essentials

» 1 tablespoon canola oil (use olive oil for a paleo version)
» Salt and ground black pepper, to taste
» 1 tablespoon butter (use olive oil for a paleo version)

DIRECTIONS

1. Add the oil and butter to a large skillet and set over medium heat. Season the fish pieces with the seafood seasoning and place in the hot pan.

2. Let them cook for 4-5 minutes per side until light golden brown. Remove from the pan and cover to keep warm.

3. In the same pan, sauté the pine nuts for 3-4 minutes.

4. Add the kale and chicken broth and cook for 3-5 minutes until the kale wilts.

5. Season with salt and pepper.

6. Place the fish on a serving dish along with sautéed kale and enjoy.

NUTRITION FACTS (PER SERVING)

Total Carbohydrates: 5g	Dietary Fiber: 1g	Net Carbs: 3g
Protein: 27g	Total Fat: 24g	Calories: 355

WHITE MEAT

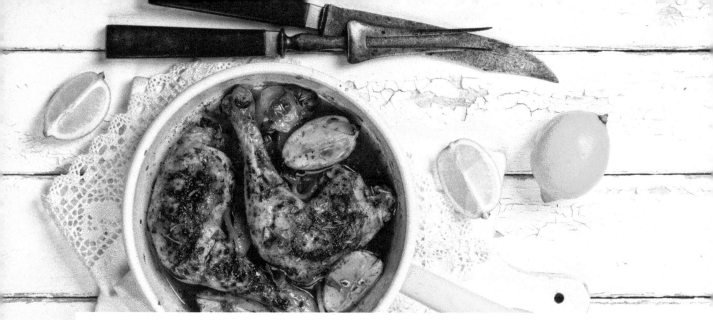

LEMONY GARLIC CHICKEN (GF)

 5 minutes   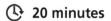 20 minutes

INGREDIENTS

» 2 chicken leg quarters (thigh and leg)
» 1 teaspoon dried basil
» 1 teaspoon dried oregano
» 2 garlic cloves, peeled and minced
» Juice and zest of ½ lemon
» 2 tablespoons fresh cilantro, chopped
» 1 tablespoon avocado oil

Essentials

» ¼ tablespoon butter (use olive oil for a paleo version)
» Salt and ground black pepper, to taste

DIRECTIONS

1. Add the avocado oil to a large skillet and set over medium heat.

2. Season the chicken with salt, pepper, basil, and oregano and place in the hot skillet.

3. Cook until browned on all sides and cooked through. Transfer to a plate and cover to keep warm.

4. In the same skillet, melt the butter.

5. Add the garlic and sauté for a minute.

6. Stir in the lemon juice. Place the drumsticks back in the skillet and spoon the juices over them. Cook for 1-2 minutes and remove from heat.

7. Place the chicken onto a serving plate, sprinkle with chopped cilantro, and serve.

NUTRITION FACTS (PER SERVING)

Total Carbohydrates: 5g	Dietary Fiber: 1g	Net Carbs: 4g
Protein: 29g	Total Fat: 15g	Calories: 270

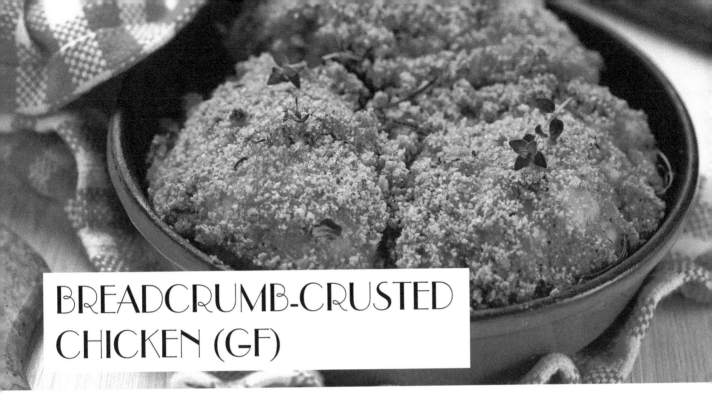

BREADCRUMB-CRUSTED CHICKEN (GF)

 10 minutes　　 **20 minutes**　　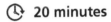

INGREDIENTS

- » ½ cup coconut flour
- » 2 boneless, skinless chicken breasts
- » ⅓ cup gluten-free almond flour breadcrumbs (use plain almond flour for a paleo version)
- » ¾ teaspoon garlic powder
- » 4 cherry tomatoes, halved
- » Small bunch of thyme leaves (removed from stalk)

Essentials

- » ⅓ cup milk (preferably soy milk) (use unsweetened almond milk for a paleo version)
- » Cooking oil spray (use coconut oil for a paleo version)
- » Salt and ground black pepper

DIRECTIONS

1. Preheat the oven to 400°F and coat a baking sheet with a little cooking oil. Set out three plates, which will be used for dipping the chicken into three different mixtures.

2. Combine the flour with ½ teaspoon salt and ½ teaspoon black pepper. Mix well and place on the first plate.

3. Pour the milk onto the second plate.

4. In a small bowl, mix the garlic powder, thyme leaves, and breadcrumbs. Add to the third plate.

5. Dip the chicken in the flour, then the milk, and then roll in the breadcrumbs mixture.

6. Once all breasts are evenly coated with all the ingredients, lay the chicken onto the prepared baking sheet, place the halved cherry tomatoes on and around the chicken breasts, and roast for 20 minutes. Before serving, ensure the chicken is golden brown and is completely cooked through.

NUTRITION FACTS (PER SERVING)

Total Carbohydrates: 15g	Dietary Fiber: 2g	Net Carbs: 13g
Protein: 25g	Total Fat: 6g	Calories: 214

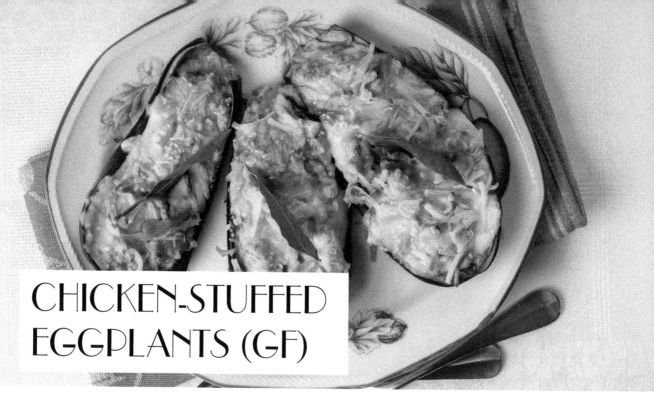

CHICKEN-STUFFED EGGPLANTS (GF)

 15 minutes   **50 minutes**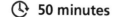

INGREDIENTS

» 1 ½ cups cooked chicken, shredded

» ¼ cup tomato-based salsa

» ¼ cup sour cream

» ¼ cup green onions, chopped

» 1 cup shredded sharp cheddar cheese + 3 tablespoons for topping (eliminate for a paleo version)

» 2 medium eggplants

Essentials

» Salt and ground black pepper, to taste

» 1 teaspoon olive oil

Optional / Garnish

» 2 tablespoons fresh parsley, chopped

DIRECTIONS

1. Preheat oven to 375°F.

2. In a bowl, mix the shredded chicken with the sour cream, salsa, 1 cup of cheddar cheese, green onion, and parsley. Stir well to combine.

3. Cut the eggplants in halves lengthwise. Prick holes in the skin using a fork. Brush them with olive oil and place in a baking dish, skin side down. Roast for about 30 minutes, until tender.

4. Remove from the oven and let them cool.

5. Scoop the flesh, being careful not to damage the skin, and combine it with the chicken mixture. Transfer the filling back to the eggplant skins and sprinkle with the remaining cheese. Return to the oven for 20 minutes until the cheese is melted and bubbly.

6. Place the eggplant halves on a serving plate and garnish with parsley, if desired.

NUTRITION FACTS (PER SERVING)

Total Carbohydrates: 8g	Dietary Fiber: 2g	Net Carbs: 6g
Protein: 30g	Total Fat: 34g	Calories: 432

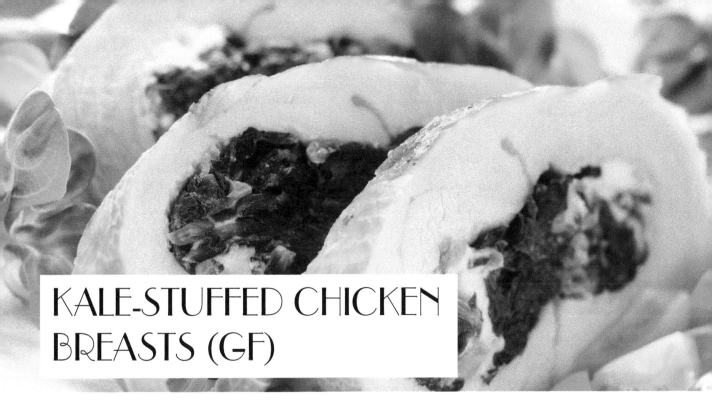

KALE-STUFFED CHICKEN BREASTS (GF)

 10 minutes   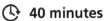 **40 minutes**

INGREDIENTS

» 2 chicken breasts, about 4 ounces each, pounded thin
» 1 egg, beaten
» ¼ cup kale leaves
» ½ cup mascarpone cheese (eliminate for a paleo version)
» ⅓ cup Parmesan cheese, grated (eliminate for a paleo version)
» ½ cup marinara sauce

Essentials

» Salt and ground black pepper to taste
» Nonstick cooking spray

DIRECTIONS

1. Preheat oven to 375°F.

2. Place the egg, kale, and mascarpone in a large bowl, and season with salt and pepper. Mix well to combine.

3. Arrange the chicken breasts on a large baking sheet coated with nonstick cooking spray.

4. Divide the cheese mixture into 2 portions and place each of them over the chicken breasts. Gently roll up. Make sure they are seam side down.

5. Spoon the marinara sauce over the chicken rolls and sprinkle with grated Parmesan cheese.

6. Bake in the oven for about 40 minutes until the cheese is melted.

NUTRITION FACTS (PER SERVING)

Total Carbohydrates: 11g	Dietary Fiber: 2g	Net Carbs: 9g
Protein: 35g	Total Fat: 25g	Calories: 422

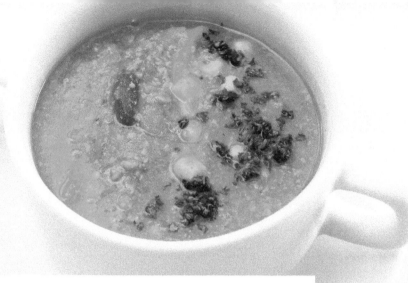

CHICKEN AND VEGETABLE SOUP (GF)

 10 minutes    **55 minutes**

INGREDIENTS

» 2 chicken legs, meat removed from the bones
» 1 small onion, peeled and chopped
» 1 small carrot, peeled and chopped
» 1 celery stalk, chopped
» 1 (14 ounce) can diced tomatoes (use fresh tomatoes for a paleo version)
» 1 (14 ounce) can vegetable broth

Essentials

» 2 tablespoons canola oil (use olive oil for a paleo version)

Optional / Garnish

» ¼ cup heavy cream (eliminate for a paleo version)
» ½ cup tinned corn

DIRECTIONS

1. Add the oil to a large nonstick skillet and set over medium-high heat.

2. Once the oil is very hot, add the chicken, and cook for 10-12 minutes, stirring frequently.

3. Stir in the carrots, celery stalk, and onion and continue cooking for another 5 minutes.

4. Add the tomatoes and vegetable broth, and bring the soup to a boil.

5. Reduce the heat, and let it simmer for about 25-30 minutes.

6. Ladle the soup into individual bowls and, if desired, top with 1-2 tablespoons of heavy cream for a delicious richness.

NUTRITION FACTS (PER SERVING)

Total Carbohydrates: 12g	Dietary Fiber: 3g	Net Carbs: 9g
Protein: 18g	Total Fat: 23g	Calories: 332

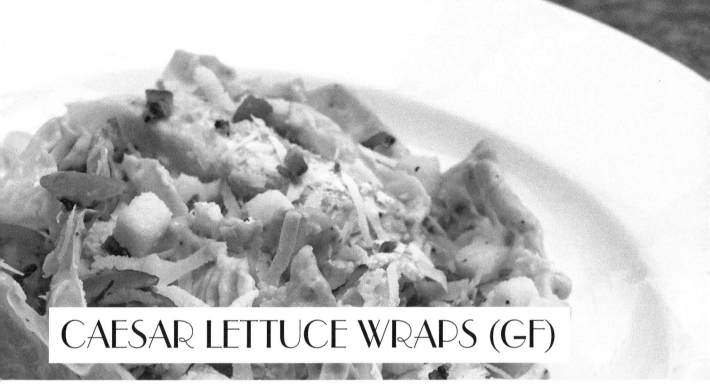

CAESAR LETTUCE WRAPS (GF)

 5 minutes   15 minutes

INGREDIENTS

» ½ head romaine lettuce
» ½ pound boneless, skinless chicken thighs
» 2 bacon strips, cooked and crumbled (be sure to use an organic and nitrate-free version for paleo)
» ½ cup cheddar cheese, shredded (eliminate for a paleo version)
» 4 tablespoons Caesar dressing (use olive oil for a paleo version)
» ½ tablespoon dried oregano

Essentials

» 1 tablespoon canola oil (use olive oil for a paleo version)

DIRECTIONS

1. Add a little oil to a large skillet and heat over medium-high heat.
2. Add the chicken and cook until golden brown on all sides and cooked through. Remove from the skillet and let it cool.
3. Chop the chicken into cubes and place in a large bowl.
4. Reserve 2 large lettuce leaves and tear or cut the remaining lettuce and add to the chicken along with the bacon crumbles and Caesar dressing. Toss well to coat.
5. Divide the salad into 2 portions and place onto reserved romaine leaves. Sprinkle the oregano generously, top with cheese, and serve.

NUTRITION FACTS (PER SERVING)

Total Carbohydrates: 8g	Dietary Fiber: 3g	Net Carbs: 5g
Protein: 46g	Total Fat: 36g	Calories: 542

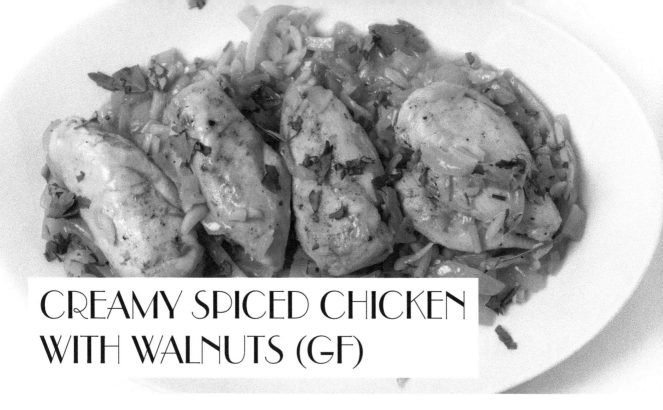

CREAMY SPICED CHICKEN WITH WALNUTS (GF)

 10 minutes   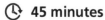 **45 minutes**

INGREDIENTS

- » 2 boneless, skinless chicken breasts
- » 2 green onions, chopped
- » 1 ½ teaspoons rosemary
- » ¼ teaspoon sage
- » 1 (10 ounce) can cream of chicken soup (be sure this is gluten-free)
- » ¼ cup walnuts, chopped

Essentials

- » ¼ cup milk

DIRECTIONS

1. Preheat oven to 375°F.

2. Arrange the chicken breasts on a rimmed baking dish. Top with the green onions.

3. In a small bowl, combine the milk, soup, rosemary, and sage. Mix well and pour over the chicken pieces.

4. Bake in the oven for 35-45 minutes. During the last 10 minutes of baking, sprinkle the chicken with the walnuts, and continue baking until the chicken is cooked through.

5. Serve alongside your favorite sautéed vegetables.

NUTRITION FACTS (PER SERVING)

Total Carbohydrates: 12g	Dietary Fiber: 2g	Net Carbs: 10g
Protein: 39g	Total Fat: 13g	Calories: 319

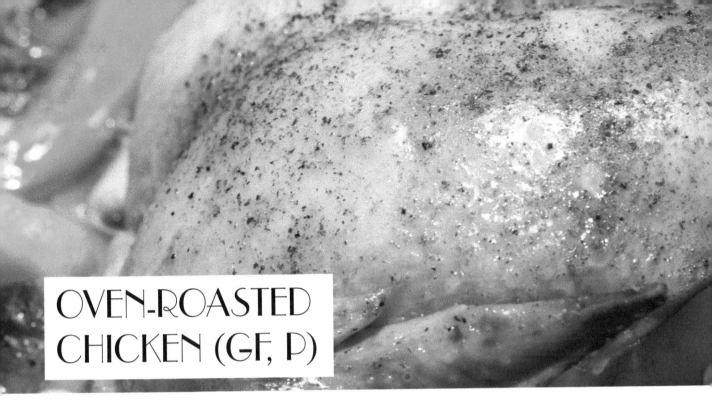

OVEN-ROASTED CHICKEN (GF, P)

 10 minutes   **1½ hours**

INGREDIENTS

- » 1 small broiler chicken (about 2 pounds)
- » ½ cup vegetable broth
- » 1 medium carrot, peeled and sliced
- » 1 medium onion, peeled and chopped
- » 1 medium zucchini, sliced
- » ½ teaspoon dried oregano

Essentials

- » Salt and pepper, to taste
- » ½ cup water

DIRECTIONS

1. Place the chicken, carrot, and onion in a large roasting pan. Season all over with salt, pepper, and dried oregano.

2. Pour the broth and water into the bottom of the roasting pan and bake in the oven, covered, until the chicken is cooked through and juices run clear, about 1½ hours. Add the zucchini 15 minutes before the cooking time is over.

3. Serve hot with the juices ladled on top.

NUTRITION FACTS (PER SERVING)

Total Carbohydrates: 9g	Dietary Fiber: 2g	Net Carbs: 7g
Protein: 33g	Total Fat: 5g	Calories: 212

29

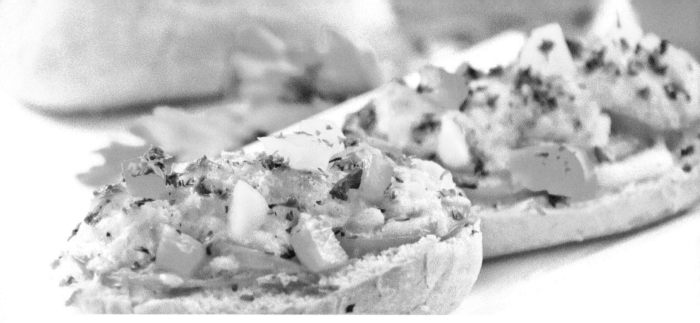

GRILLED BRUSCHETTA (GF)

 15 minutes **5 minutes**   👥

INGREDIENTS

- » 2 medium ripe tomatoes
- » 1 garlic clove, peeled and minced
- » ¼ cup yellow onion, peeled and chopped
- » 1 tablespoon fresh basil, chopped
- » 3 ounces cheddar cheese, diced (eliminate for a paleo version)
- » 2 chicken cutlets, sliced thin

Vegetarian option

- » 2 pieces low-carb bread.

Essentials

- » 1 tablespoon canola oil (use olive oil for a paleo version)
- » Salt and ground black pepper, to taste
- » 1 tablespoon balsamic vinegar

DIRECTIONS

1. Wash the tomatoes, chop them into small cubes, and place in a bowl.

2. Add the onion, garlic, sunflower oil, balsamic vinegar, salt, and pepper to taste. Mix to combine and let the mixture sit for 15-30 minutes to allow the flavors to blend.

3. Season the chicken with salt and black pepper.

4. Preheat the grill to medium-high. Coat the grill grates with oil.

5. Grill the chicken cutlets for about 2-4 minutes per side, until golden and cooked through. Transfer to a serving plate.

6. Spoon the tomato mixture over the top of grilled cutlets and serve. As a vegetarian alternative, use low-carb bread instead of chicken.

7. Top with cheese and grill for about 30 seconds until the cheese begins to melt. Sprinkle over the chopped basil and serve hot or cold.

NUTRITION FACTS (PER SERVING)

Total Carbohydrates: 14g	Dietary Fiber: 4g	Net Carbs: 10g
Protein: 36g	Total Fat: 15g	Calories: 348

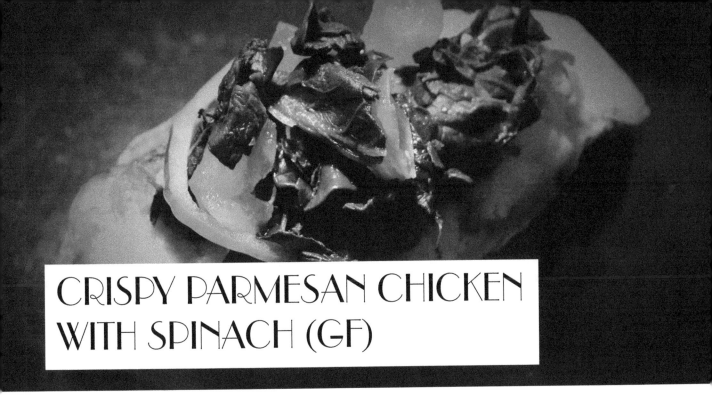

CRISPY PARMESAN CHICKEN WITH SPINACH (GF)

 10 minutes   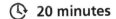 **20 minutes**

INGREDIENTS

» 2 medium chicken breasts (about 4 ounces each)
» 2 green onions, chopped
» 4 ounces frozen spinach, thawed and drained
» 2 ounces Parmesan cheese, grated (eliminate for a paleo version)
» ½ cup roasted bell pepper, sliced in strips

Essentials

» Salt and ground black pepper, to taste
» 1 teaspoon olive oil

DIRECTIONS

1. Preheat oven to 400°F.

2. Using a sharp knife, slice the chicken breasts lengthwise to make 4 cutlets and season with salt and pepper.

3. Grill the chicken for about 8 minutes, until lightly golden on both sides. Be careful not to overcook, but ensure the chicken is not pink on the inside.

4. Add the oil to a large skillet and set over medium heat. Add the green onions and cook for a minute, stirring frequently.

5. Add the spinach, season with salt and pepper and cook for 3-5 minutes until the greens wilt.

6. Line a baking sheet with aluminum foil. Arrange grilled chicken cutlets on it. Top with sautéed spinach followed by the grated Parmesan cheese and roasted pepper slices. Bake for 6-8 minutes, until the cheese is melted and bubbly.

7. Serve hot.

NUTRITION FACTS (PER SERVING)

Total Carbohydrates: 6g	Dietary Fiber: 1g	Net Carbs: 5g
Protein: 43g	Total Fat: 20g	Calories: 328

RED MEAT

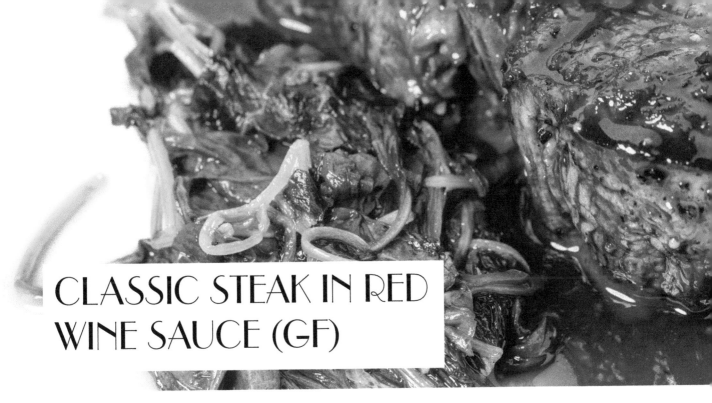

CLASSIC STEAK IN RED WINE SAUCE (GF)

 15 minutes   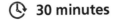 **30 minutes**

INGREDIENTS

- » ½ pound sirloin steak (about 1¼-inch thick) or venison steak
- » 4 ounces white mushrooms, cleaned, trimmed, and sliced
- » 1 cup vegetable stock
- » ½ cup dry red wine
- » 2 green onions, chopped
- » 2 cups baby spinach leaves

Essentials

- » 2 teaspoons coconut oil, for cooking
- » Salt and ground black pepper, to taste

DIRECTIONS

1. Place a large cast-iron pan over medium-high heat.
2. Place the steak in the hot pan. Brown on both sides, about 4-5 minutes per side. Season with salt and pepper while cooking. Transfer to a plate and cover to keep warm.
3. In the same pan heat the coconut oil. Add the mushrooms and sauté for 3-4 minutes. Remove from the pan.
4. Increase the heat to high. Add the green onions, wine, and stock to the pan and bring the mixture to a boil. Season with salt and pepper. Once the pan content has reduced to ½ cup, turn off the heat.
5. Add a little oil to another pan and sauté the spinach on a medium-high heat for 1-2 minutes until they wilt. Place the spinach in a large bowl. Take 4 tablespoons of wine mixture and drizzle over the spinach. Mix well.
6. Divide the spinach among 2 serving plates. Put the steak, either sliced or whole, and mushrooms on the top, spoon the remaining wine mixture over, and serve.

NUTRITION FACTS (PER SERVING)

Total Carbohydrates: 14g	Dietary Fiber: 5g	Net Carbs: 9g
Protein: 28g	Total Fat: 18g	Calories: 338

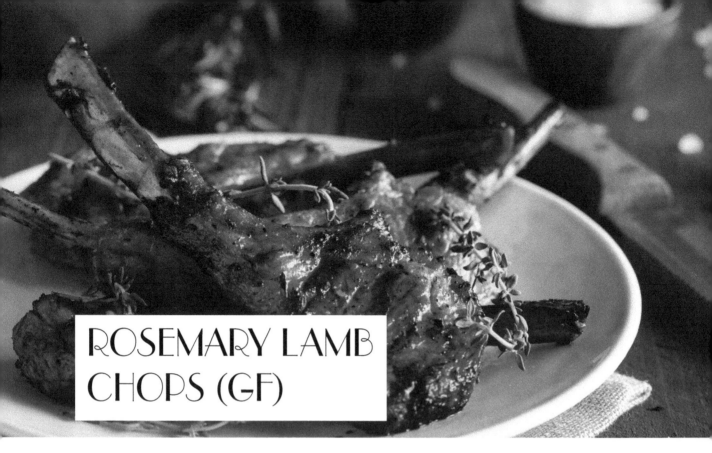

ROSEMARY LAMB CHOPS (GF)

 10 minutes   **25 minutes**

INGREDIENTS

» 4 lamb chops
» 2 teaspoons fresh rosemary

Essentials

» 1 tablespoons extra virgin olive oil
» 1 tablespoon butter (use extra olive oil for a paleo version) Optional
» Fresh garlic, to taste
» Salt and ground black pepper, to taste

DIRECTIONS

1. Add the butter and olive oil to a large skillet and place over medium-high heat.

2. Place the lamb chops in the hot skillet and cook for 2-3 minutes and flip.

3. Sprinkle the top side with ¾ of the fresh rosemary and cook for 7-8 minutes, then flip to brown the other side as well.

4. Once the chops are golden brown, reduce the heat to low and cook for another 4-5 minutes until they are cooked through.

5. Place on a serving plate, garnish with the remaining rosemary, and serve.

NUTRITION FACTS (PER SERVING)

Total Carbohydrates: 0g	Dietary Fiber: 0g	Net Carbs: 0g
Protein: 16g	Total Fat: 15g	Calories: 198

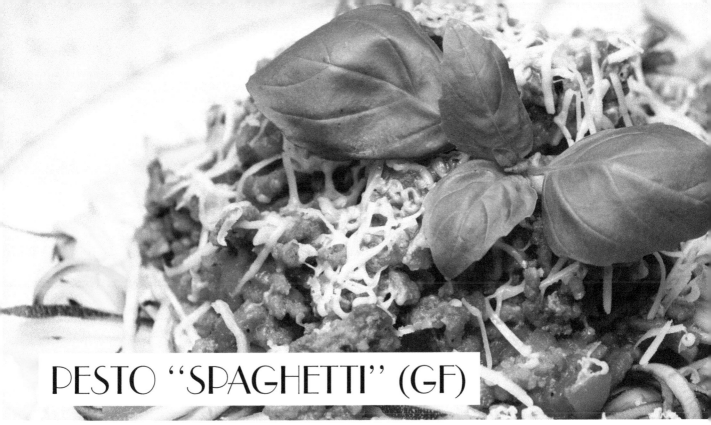

PESTO "SPAGHETTI" (GF)

 5 minutes   **25 minutes**

INGREDIENTS:

- » ½ pound ground round
- » ¼ cup basil pesto (be sure this is gluten-free)
- » Bunch of fresh basil, chopped
- » ¼ cup shredded mozzarella cheese (eliminate for a paleo version)
- » 2 medium zucchini
- » 6 cherry tomatoes, chopped

Essentials

- » 2 tablespoons coconut oil, for cooking, divided

DIRECTIONS:

1. Melt 1 tablespoon coconut oil in a saucepan over medium-high heat.

2. Add ground beef and cook for about 5-8 minutes until brown, stirring frequently.

3. Stir in the pesto, tomatoes and fresh chopped basil. Reduce the heat to low and cook for at least 2 minutes. Turn off the heat and transfer the ground beef mixture to a bowl.

4. To make zucchini noodles, pass the zucchini through a spiralizer.

5. Heat the remaining 1 tablespoon of coconut oil in a saucepan over medium-high heat. Add the zoodles (zucchini noodles) and sauté for 3-4 minutes or until al dente. Make sure not to overcook.

6. Add the zoodles to the ground beef mixture and mix well to combine. Top with grated mozzarella cheese.

7. Divide onto 2 plates and serve immediately.

NUTRITION FACTS (PER SERVING)

Total Carbohydrates: 2g	**Dietary Fiber: 1g**	**Net Carbs: 1g**
Protein: 29g	**Total Fat: 45g**	**Calories: 521**

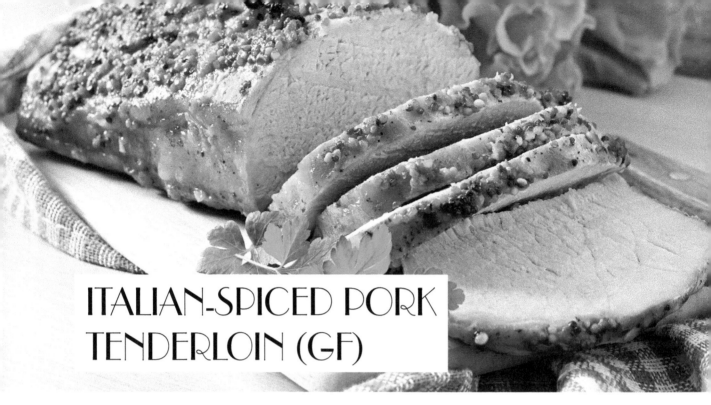

ITALIAN-SPICED PORK TENDERLOIN (GF)

 10 minutes   **30 minutes**

INGREDIENTS

- » 1 teaspoon dried oregano
- » 1 onion, peeled and diced
- » 1 slice gluten-free bread (use ½ cup of almond flour for a paleo version)
- » 1 garlic clove, peeled and minced
- » 1 large egg white, beaten
- » ½ pound pork tenderloin, trimmed of excess fat

Essentials

- » Salt and ground black pepper, to taste
- » Cooking spray (use coconut oil for a paleo version)

DIRECTIONS

1. Preheat the oven to 400°F. Spray a broiler pan with cooking oil spray.
2. Combine the oregano, onion, garlic, and bread in a food processor and process until finely ground. You should have about ⅓ cup breadcrumbs.
3. Transfer the breadcrumbs to a plate.
4. Season the pork with salt and black pepper.
5. Dip the meat into the beaten egg white, and then roll in the bread crumb mixture until coated evenly.
6. Place the pork on the broiler pan and roast for about 20 minutes. Remove from the oven and let rest for 5 minutes.
7. Cut the pork into ¼-inch thick slices and serve.

NUTRITION FACTS (PER SERVING)

Total Carbohydrates: 13g	Dietary Fiber: 2g	Net Carbs: 11g
Protein: 34g	Total Fat: 5g	Calories: 232

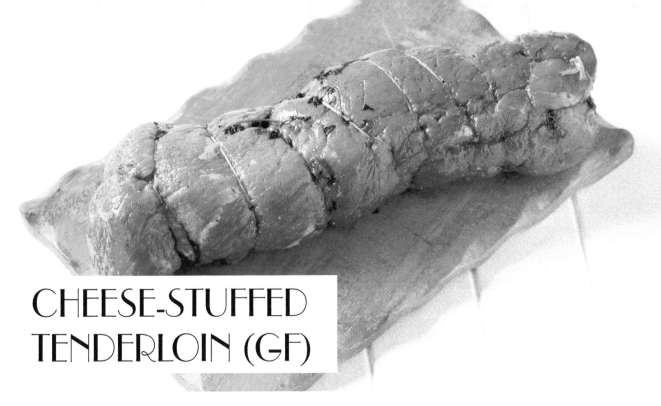

CHEESE-STUFFED TENDERLOIN (GF)

 15 minutes   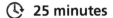 **25 minutes**

INGREDIENTS

- » ½ pound pork tenderloin
- » 2 tablespoons grated Pecorino cheese
- » 2 tablespoons crumbled feta cheese
- » 1 green onion, chopped
- » 1 tablespoon cashews, finely crushed
- » ½ teaspoon onion, diced

Essentials

- » Salt and ground black pepper, to taste

DIRECTIONS

1. Preheat grill.

2. Using a sharp knife, cut a pocket, running lengthwise, into the pork tenderloin.

3. Place the green onion, onions, crushed cashews, Pecorino cheese, and feta cheese in a medium bowl and mix well to combine.

4. Spoon the mixture into the pocket and secure the pocket with a skewer or wrap in butcher's twine.

5. Sprinkle the pork with salt and freshly ground pepper and grill until golden brown and juices run clear.

NUTRITION FACTS (PER SERVING)

Total Carbohydrates: 14g	Dietary Fiber: 4g	Net Carbs: 10g
Protein: 36g	Total Fat: 13g	Calories: 320

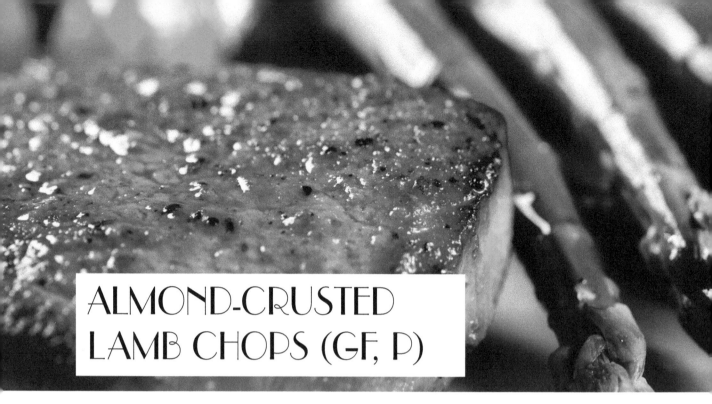

ALMOND-CRUSTED LAMB CHOPS (GF, P)

 10 minutes   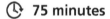 75 minutes

INGREDIENTS

» 2 lamb chops, 1-inch thick
» 2 teaspoons Dijon mustard
» ½ cup ground almonds
» 10 asparagus spears, trimmed
» 4 cherry tomatoes

Essentials

» Salt and ground black pepper, to taste

DIRECTIONS

1. Preheat oven to 350°F.

2. Season the lamb chops on both sides with salt and pepper.

3. Coat the chops with mustard and sprinkle with ground almonds until covered. Reserve a bit of the almonds for the vegetables.

4. Arrange the lamb chops in a roasting pan and roast for about 50-60 minutes until they acquire a golden crust.

5. Coat the asparagus and cherry tomatoes with a little oil, and then sprinkle the remaining ground almonds over the vegetables. Roast next to the chops for about 15 minutes.

6. Remove everything from the oven and serve hot.

NUTRITION FACTS (PER SERVING)

Total Carbohydrates: 10g	Dietary Fiber: 4g	Net Carbs: 6g
Protein: 15g	Total Fat: 14g	Calories: 219

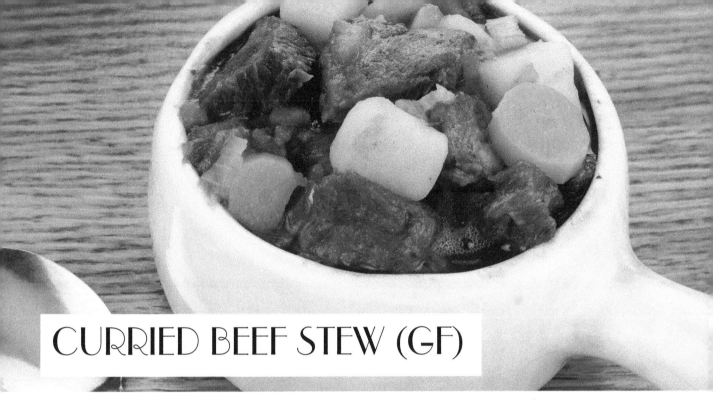

CURRIED BEEF STEW (GF)

 20 minutes   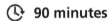 **90 minutes**

INGREDIENTS

- » ¾ pound beef stew meat
- » 1 ½ cups vegetable stock
- » 1 small red onion, peeled and chopped
- » 2 garlic cloves, peeled and minced
- » 1 medium carrot, peeled and sliced
- » 1 medium turnip, peeled and cut into chunks

Essentials

- » Salt and ground black pepper, to taste
- » ⅔ teaspoon curry powder
- » 1 tablespoon canola oil (use olive oil for a paleo version)

DIRECTIONS

1. Season the meat with salt and pepper and toss with hands to coat.

2. Heat the oil in a large stockpot over medium heat. Add the meat and brown on both sides.

3. Add the onion and garlic and cook for a minute. Then, add the vegetable stock and curry powder. Once the mixture begins to boil, reduce the heat to medium-low, cover, and let it simmer for about 1 hour, putting in the turnip chunks after 30 minutes.

4. Add the carrots and continue cooking for another 30 minutes until the vegetables are tender and the meat is cooked through.

NUTRITION FACTS (PER SERVING)

Total Carbohydrates: 10g	Dietary Fiber: 2g	Net Carbs: 8g
Protein: 50g	Total Fat: 29g	Calories: 531

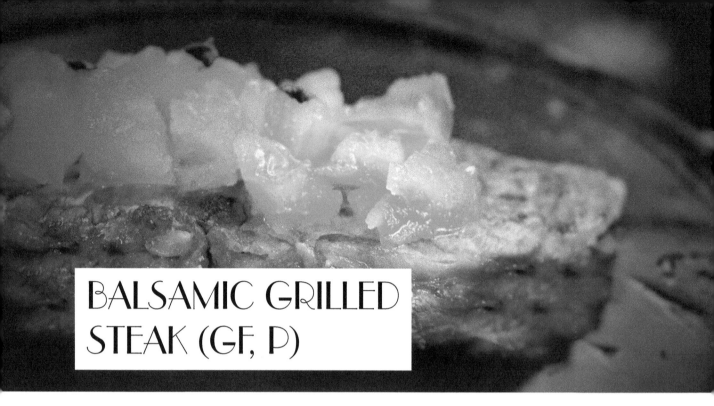

BALSAMIC GRILLED STEAK (GF, P)

 30 minutes   🕐 15 minutes   👤👤👤👤

INGREDIENTS

» 1 pound flank steak, trimmed of excess fat
» 1 tablespoon balsamic vinegar
» ¼ cup red onion, chopped
» teaspoon garlic powder
» 2-3 tomatoes, chopped (about 3 ½ cups)
» ½ tablespoon fresh basil or parsley

Essentials

» 1 tablespoon extra virgin olive oil
» Salt and freshly ground black pepper

DIRECTIONS

1. Using a fork, pierce the steak in several places and sprinkle with garlic powder, salt, and pepper. Rub with your hands and allow to rest for 15 minutes at room temperature.

2. Add the onions, olive oil, and vinegar to a large bowl, season with salt and pepper, and mix to combine. Let the mixture sit for 5 minutes.

3. Add the tomatoes and herbs to the bowl. Mix well.

4. Heat a broiler or grill to high heat. Grill the steak about 8 minutes per side or to your desired doneness.

5. Transfer to a plate and let it cool for 5 minutes before slicing. Using a sharp knife, slice the steak thin, top with the tomato mixture, and enjoy.

NUTRITION FACTS (PER SERVING)

Total Carbohydrates: 5g	Dietary Fiber: 1g	Net Carbs: 4g
Protein: 18g	Total Fat: 8g	Calories: 170

VEGETERIAN

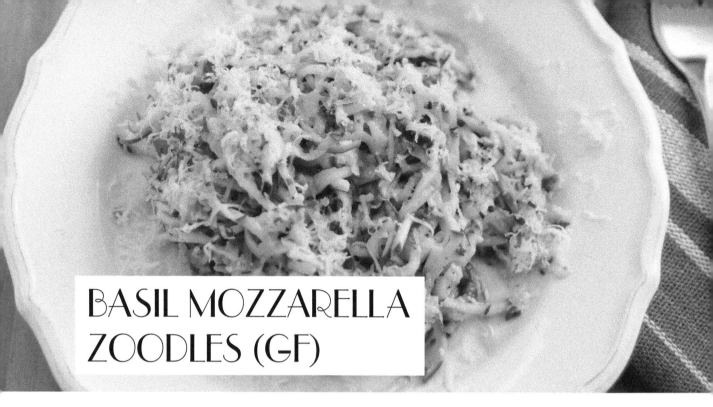

BASIL MOZZARELLA ZOODLES (GF)

 10 minutes   10 minutes

INGREDIENTS

» 3 medium zucchinis, spiralized
» Small bunch of basil leaves
» ½ teaspoon garlic powder
» 1 tablespoon pine nuts, toasted
» 2 tablespoons fresh lemon juice
» ¼ cup shredded mozzarella cheese (eliminate for a paleo version)

Essentials

» 1 tablespoon canola oil (use olive oil for a paleo version)
» Salt and ground black pepper, to taste

DIRECTIONS

1. Add the olive oil to a large pan and set over medium heat.
2. Add the zoodles and sauté for a few minutes until light golden and al dente.
3. Season with the garlic powder, salt, and pepper.
4. Add the basil leaves, pine nuts, and lemon juice and reduce heat to low. Simmer for 2-4 minutes. When sauce thickens to your liking, sprinkle with mozzarella cheese and remove from heat.
5. Serve warm.

NUTRITION FACTS (PER SERVING)

Total Carbohydrates: 5g	Dietary Fiber: 1g	Net Carbs: 4g
Protein: 6g	Total Fat: 7g	Calories: 101

42

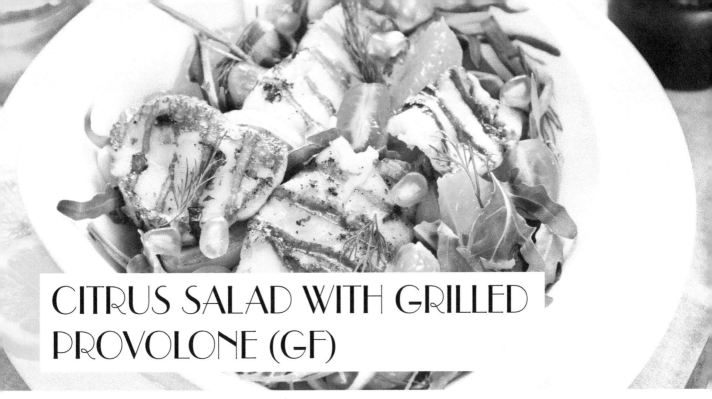

CITRUS SALAD WITH GRILLED PROVOLONE (GF)

 15 minutes 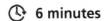 **6 minutes**

INGREDIENTS

- » 2 cups arugula
- » 2 clementines, peeled and segmented
- » 3 ounces provolone cheese (eliminate for a paleo version)
- » 5 cherry tomatoes, halved
- » ½ pomegranate, deseeded
- » 1 teaspoon lemon juice

Essentials

- » Sea salt, to taste
- » 2 teaspoons olive oil

DIRECTIONS

1. Slice the provolone cheese into thick, bite-size pieces.
2. Place the cheese pieces on a preheated grill for about 3 minutes on each side. Grill marks should appear on the cheese.
3. Place the arugula into a large salad bowl and toss with the clementines, cherry tomatoes, and pomegranate seeds.
4. Top the salad with the beautifully grilled provolone slices.
5. In a small bowl, mix the olive oil, lemon juice, and salt.
6. Drizzle this mixture over the salad.

NUTRITION FACTS (PER SERVING)

Total Carbohydrates: 14g	Dietary Fiber: 5g	Net Carbs: 9g
Protein: 13g	Total Fat: 17g	Calories: 256

43

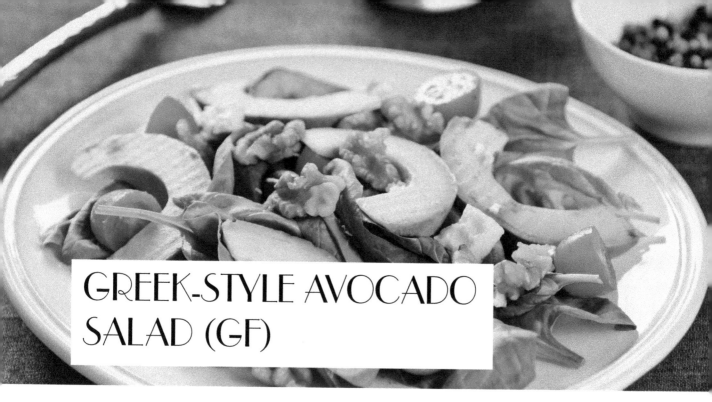

GREEK-STYLE AVOCADO SALAD (GF)

 5 minutes   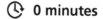 **0 minutes**

INGREDIENTS

- » 1 large avocado, pitted and flesh removed
- » 3 Roma tomatoes
- » ½ cup crushed walnuts
- » 1 cup feta cheese, crumbled (eliminate for a paleo version)
- » 2 garlic cloves, peeled and minced
- » 2 cups fresh basil leaves or baby spinach

Essentials

- » 2 tablespoons olive oil
- » 1 tablespoon lemon juice
- » Salt and pepper to taste

DIRECTIONS

1. Chop the avocado into about ½ inch chunks. Transfer to a serving bowl.
2. Slice the tomatoes and add to the bowl with the walnuts.
3. In a small bowl, whisk the olive oil, lemon juice, and garlic together.
4. Crumble the feta cheese into the bowl, drizzle with the dressing, and toss until everything is well combined.
5. Serve on a bed of basil leaves or baby spinach.
6. Season with salt and black pepper to taste.

NUTRITION FACTS (PER SERVING)

Total Carbohydrates: 18g	Dietary Fiber: 9g	Net Carbs: 9g
Protein: 7g	Total Fat: 32g	Calories: 371

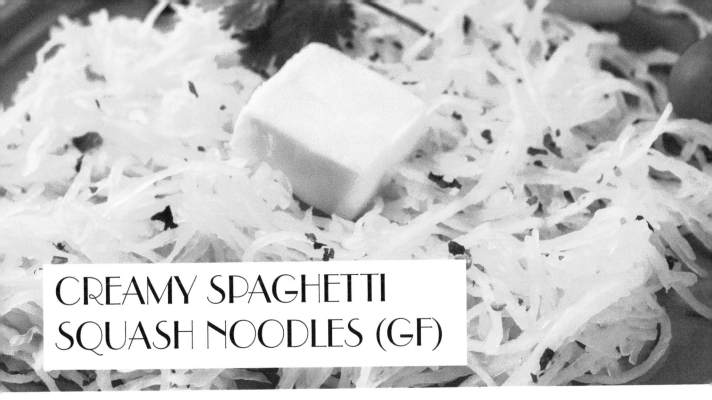

CREAMY SPAGHETTI SQUASH NOODLES (GF)

 15 minutes   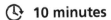 **10 minutes**

INGREDIENTS

» 1 medium spaghetti squash
» ¼ cup feta cheese, crumbled
» 3 tablespoons heavy cream
» Juice of ½ a lemon
» Small bunch of fresh basil, chopped

Essentials

» 2 tablespoons olive oil
» Salt and ground black pepper, to taste

Optional

» Italian seasoning
» Garlic powder
» 1 tablespoon butter

DIRECTIONS

1. Preheat oven to 375°F. Slice the spaghetti squash in half lengthwise and use a spoon to scrape out the seeds. Coat the inside of each half with a little olive oil, place on a baking tray (skin side up), and bake for about 40 minutes. At this point, you should be able to pierce the squash easily. Allow to cool slightly.

2. Use a fork to pull the inside flesh into strands. Transfer the strands into a serving bowl and discard the remaining squash.

3. In a small bowl, whisk together the heavy cream, lemon juice, and chopped basil. Mix until well combined.

4. Add the feta cheese to the squash noodles, season with salt and pepper, and mix well.

5. Drizzle the squash noodles with the heavy cream mixture. Mix until the noodles are fully coated with the sauce.

6. Divide between two plates, top with a pat of butter, if desired, and serve.

NUTRITION FACTS (PER SERVING)

Total Carbohydrates: 12g   Dietary Fiber: 3g   Net Carbs: 9g
Protein: 5g   Total Fat: 33g   Calories: 339

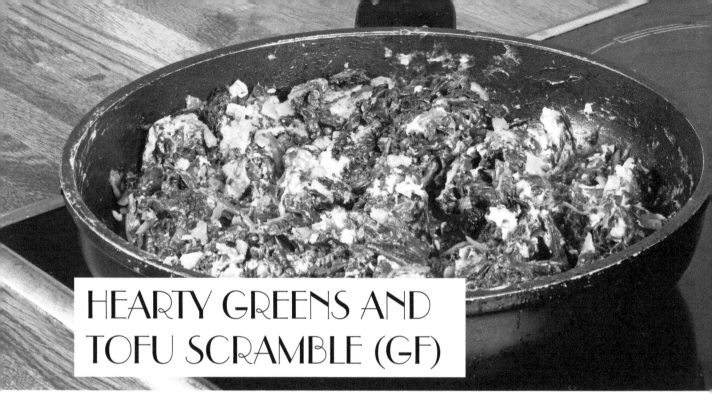

HEARTY GREENS AND TOFU SCRAMBLE (GF)

 20 minutes   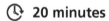 **20 minutes**

INGREDIENTS

- » ½ large head cabbage, thinly sliced
- » ½ red onion, peeled and sliced
- » 2 large handfuls baby spinach
- » 2 garlic cloves, peeled and minced
- » 8 ounces extra-firm tofu
- » 12 Kalamata olives

Essentials

- » 2 tablespoons olive oil
- » Salt and ground black pepper, to taste

DIRECTIONS

1. Wrap the tofu in cheesecloth and top with a teapot or cast-iron pan to press the excess liquid out.

2. In a large bowl, combine the cabbage, onion, garlic, and 1 tablespoon olive oil. Season with salt and pepper and mix well to coat.

3. Heat the remaining olive oil in a large skillet over medium heat.

4. Add the cabbage mixture to the skillet and sauté for 5-7 minutes until the cabbage is slightly tender.

5. Add the spinach to the pan and reduce heat to low.

6. Using a fork, crumble the tofu into the skillet. Add the Kalamata olives and mix well to combine.

7. Cook for 10-12 minutes until the tofu is golden brown and the spinach and cabbage are tender.

8. Season with salt and pepper, divide between two plates, and serve.

NUTRITION FACTS (PER SERVING)

Total Carbohydrates: 6g	Dietary Fiber: 1g	Net Carbs: 5g
Protein: 12g	Total Fat: 23g	Calories: 260

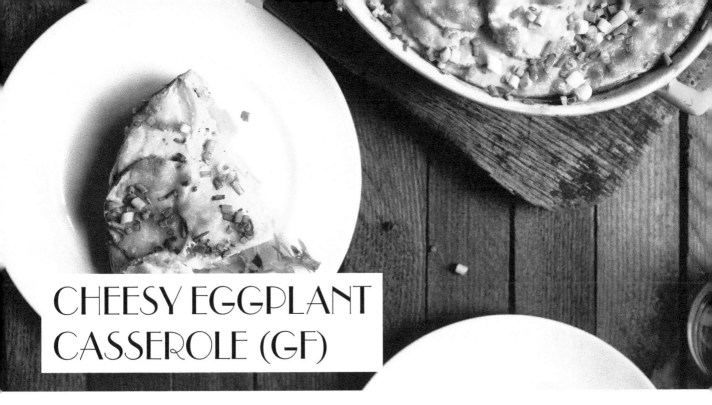

CHEESY EGGPLANT CASSEROLE (GF)

 30 minutes   **45 minutes**

INGREDIENTS

- » 2 small eggplants, sliced about ¼-inch thick
- » ½ red bell pepper, seeded and diced
- » ¼ cup gluten-free bran flakes or gluten-free breadcrumbs (use almond flour for a paleo version)
- » ½ cup shredded mozzarella cheese (eliminate for a paleo version)
- » 1 cup kale, chopped
- » 1 egg, beaten

Essentials

- » ¼ cup olive oil
- » Salt and ground black pepper to taste

DIRECTIONS

1. Preheat oven to 350°F.

2. Coat an 8-in by 8-inch baking dish with oil.

3. Place the bell pepper, sliced eggplant, cheese, egg, bran flakes, and kale in a bowl.

4. Drizzle with oil and season with salt and pepper. Mix well to coat and transfer to the prepared baking dish. Spread in an even layer and bake in the oven for 40 minutes until the vegetables are tender and the top is golden brown.

5. Serve immediately.

NUTRITION FACTS (PER SERVING)

| Total Carbohydrates: 21g | Dietary Fiber: 10g | Net Carbs: 11g |
| Protein: 16g | Total Fat: 14g | Calories: 311 |

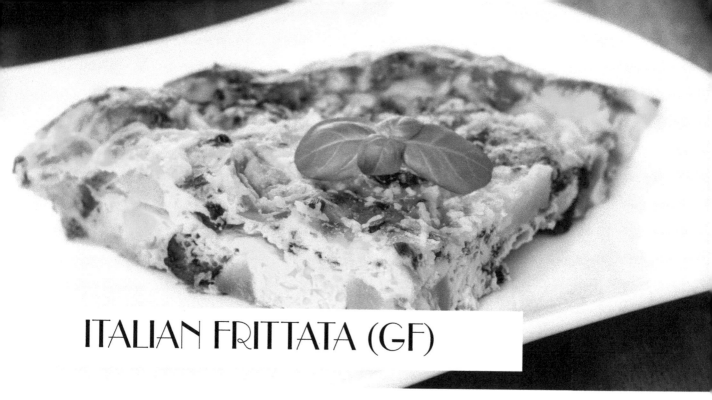

ITALIAN FRITTATA (GF)

 10 minutes   **10 minutes**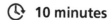

INGREDIENTS

» 1 ½ cups fresh cauliflower florets
» 1 bell pepper, seeded and julienned
» 1 teaspoon garlic powder
» 4 cherry tomatoes, halved
» 1 tablespoon goat cheese, crumbled (eliminate for a paleo version)
» 4 medium eggs

Essentials

» 1 tablespoon canola oil (use olive oil for a paleo version)
» Salt and ground black pepper, to taste
» ⅔ teaspoon dried thyme
» ½ cup milk (use unsweetened almond milk or full-fat coconut milk for a paleo version)

DIRECTIONS

1. Preheat oven to 350°F.
2. Place the cauliflower florets in a large pot of boiling water. Cook for 3-4 minutes until crisp-tender. Transfer to a colander and drain.
3. In a large pan, heat the oil over medium heat. Add the julienned peppers and sauté for 3-4 minutes. Make sure not to overcook.
4. Add the cauliflower and garlic powder to the pan. Season with thyme, salt, and pepper, and cook for 1-2 minutes.
5. Stir in the tomatoes and cook until heated through.
6. Beat the eggs and milk together until frothy. Pour the egg mixture evenly across the pan. Cook for about 2 minutes until a small crust is formed on the bottom. Use a spatula to ease the egg slightly away from the pan and continue to cook for another 3-4 minutes, until the bottom is golden.
7. Sprinkle the crumbled goat cheese over the frittata and place in the oven for 6-8 minutes.
8. Remove from the oven and let it stand for 5 minutes covered. Slice into wedges and serve warm.

NUTRITION FACTS (PER SERVING)

Total Carbohydrates: 12g	Dietary Fiber: 5g	Net Carbs: 7g
Protein: 16g	Total Fat: 18g	Calories: 258

48

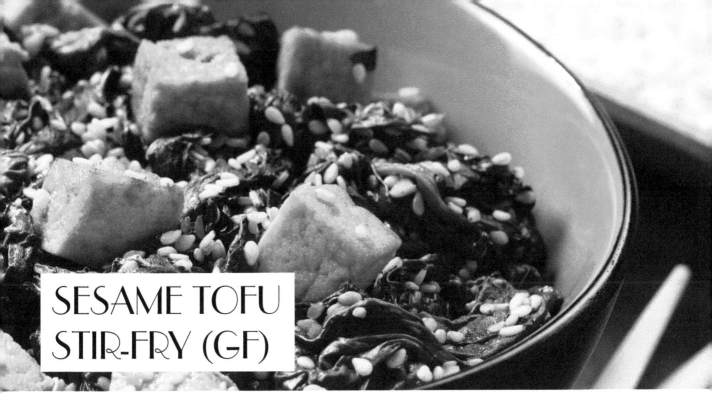

SESAME TOFU STIR-FRY (GF)

 20 minutes   **15 minutes**

INGREDIENTS

- » 8 ounces extra firm tofu, pressed dry
- » 1 teaspoon minced fresh ginger
- » 1 cup kale, chopped
- » ½ teaspoon garlic powder
- » 2-3 tablespoons gluten-free soy sauce, to taste
- » 2 tablespoons toasted sesame seeds

Essentials

- » 1 tablespoon sesame oil

DIRECTIONS

1. Cut the tofu into small cubes, about ½ inch
2. Add the sesame oil to a large skillet and place over medium-high heat.
3. Add the tofu and sauté until golden on all sides.
4. Add the fresh ginger, kale, and desired amount of soy sauce. Cook for 3-5 minutes, stirring frequently, until the kale wilts.
5. Remove from heat and divide into 2 serving bowls. Top with sesame seeds and serve.

NUTRITION FACTS (PER SERVING)

Total Carbohydrates: 7g	Dietary Fiber: 2g	Net Carbs: 5g
Protein: 15g	Total Fat: 17g	Calories: 226

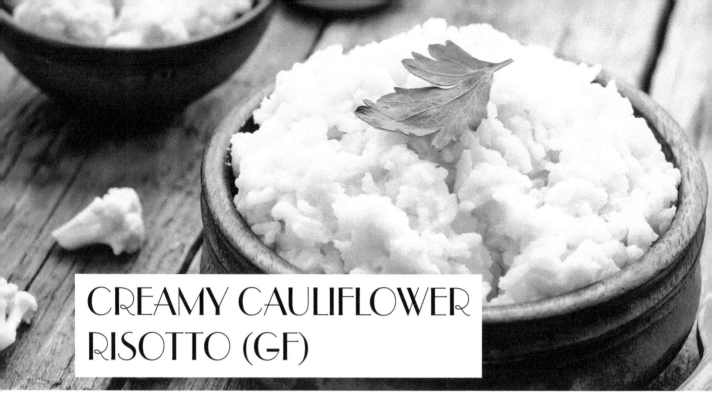

CREAMY CAULIFLOWER RISOTTO (GF)

 10 minutes   **10 minutes**   👥

INGREDIENTS

» 2 cups cauliflower
» 8 medium white button mushrooms, trimmed
» 3 garlic cloves, peeled and minced
» 1 cup vegetable broth
» ½ cup cream cheese
» ½ cup mozzarella cheese

Essentials

» 2 tablespoons olive oil
» Salt and ground black pepper, to taste
» 1 teaspoon dried oregano

DIRECTIONS

1. Thoroughly wash the cauliflower, cut into florets, and place in a food processor.
2. Pulse for 1-2 minutes, until it resembles white rice. Alternatively, you can use a box grater to achieve the same result.
3. Add 1 tablespoon of olive oil to a medium saucepan and set over medium heat. Add the garlic and mushrooms and sauté for about 2 minutes.
4. Add the "cauliflower rice", give a stir and pour in the vegetable broth.
5. Bring the mixture to a simmer and reduce heat to low. Cover and cook for 5 minutes, stirring 1-2 times. When the cauliflower is al dente, remove the lid, and continue cooking for another 7-10 minutes until all the liquid has been absorbed. Watch closely so it does not begin to burn.
6. Stir in the cream cheese and mozzarella cheese and season with salt, pepper, and oregano. Stir well.
7. Once the cheese is melted, remove the saucepan from the heat.
8. Transfer to a serving bowl and serve warm.

NUTRITION FACTS (PER SERVING)

Total Carbohydrates: 12g	Dietary Fiber: 4g	Net Carbs: 8g
Protein: 18g	Total Fat: 34g	Calories: 423

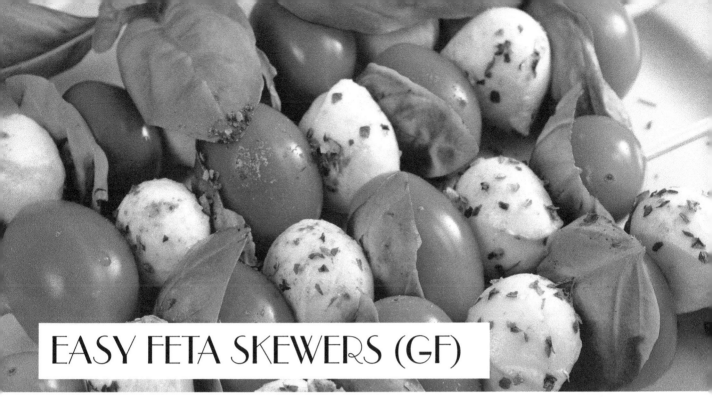

EASY FETA SKEWERS (GF)

 10 minutes 0 minutes

INGREDIENTS

- » 2 cups cherry tomatoes
- » 1 cup fresh basil leaves
- » 2 cups baby mozzarella cheese balls
- » 1 tablespoon oregano
- » 1-2 tablespoons extra virgin olive oil

Optional

- » 1 cup yellow bell pepper (these can add a nice crunch to the skewers)

DIRECTIONS

1. Wash the cherry tomatoes, bell peppers, and basil.
2. Chop the bell pepper in small squares.
3. Combine the olive oil with the oregano and rub the mozzarella balls with this mixture.
4. Carefully assemble the ingredients on skewers in the following order: tomatoes, mozzarella, bell pepper, and basil leaves and serve.

NUTRITION FACTS (PER SERVING)

Total Carbohydrates: 9g	Dietary Fiber: 2g	Net Carbs: 7g
Protein: 13g	Total Fat: 22g	Calories: 280

SIDE DISHES/SNACKS

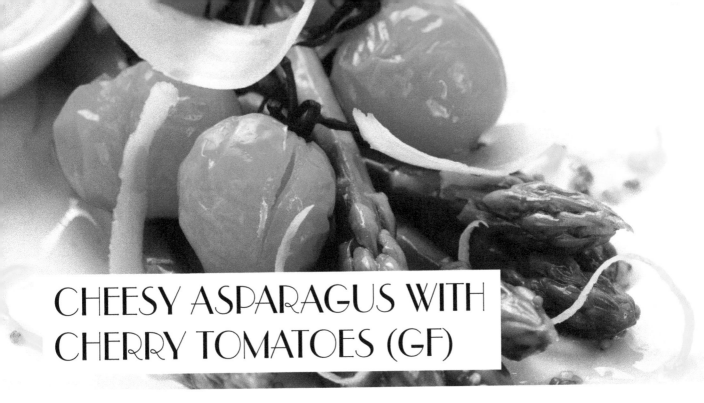

CHEESY ASPARAGUS WITH CHERRY TOMATOES (GF)

 5 minutes   12 minutes

INGREDIENTS

» 1 small bunch fresh asparagus, trimmed
» ¼ cup Romano cheese, grated (eliminate for a paleo version)
» 1 onion, peeled and sliced thin
» 2 garlic cloves, peeled and minced
» 10 cherry tomatoes, halved

Essentials

» ¼ cup extra virgin olive oil
» ⅔ cup water

DIRECTIONS

1. Add the water and asparagus to a large skillet and set over medium heat.

2. Cook about 10 minutes until the asparagus softens. Drain water from the pan and return to the stove over low heat.

3. Add the olive oil, onion, garlic, and tomatoes to the asparagus and mix well to combine. Top with grated cheese and cook for another 1-2 minutes until the cheese is melted.

NUTRITION FACTS (PER SERVING)

Total Carbohydrates: 9g	Dietary Fiber: 2g	Net Carbs: 7g
Protein: 5g	Total Fat: 15g	Calories: 193

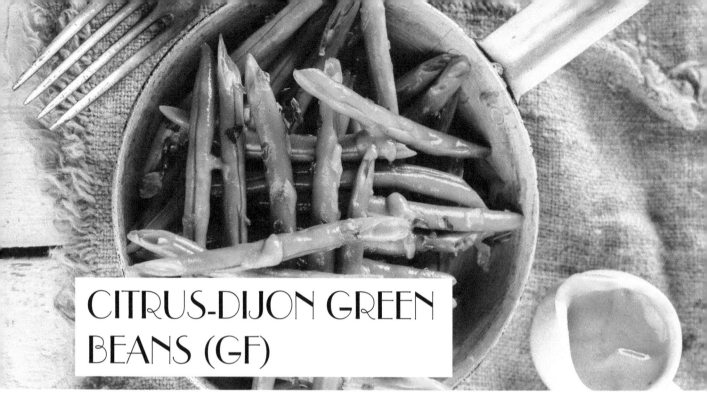

CITRUS-DIJON GREEN BEANS (GF)

 10 minutes 10 minutes

INGREDIENTS

- » ½ pound French green beans, trimmed
- » 1 lime, juiced
- » 1 tablespoon Dijon mustard
- » 2 garlic cloves, peeled and minced
- » 2 tablespoons heavy cream (eliminate for a paleo version)

Essentials

- » 1 tablespoon butter (use olive oil for a paleo version)

DIRECTIONS

1. Add the green beans to a pot of boiling water and cook for about 5 minutes until crisp-tender.

2. Meanwhile, melt the butter in a medium skillet over medium heat. Add the garlic and cook for 1 minute.

3. Stir in the heavy cream and mustard. Cook for another 3-4 minutes.

4. Drain the green beans and add to the mustard mixture.

5. Add the lime juice and stir well to combine.

6. Serve immediately. The mustard flavor pairs well with a red meat dish.

NUTRITION FACTS (PER SERVING)

Total Carbohydrates: 12g	Dietary Fiber: 4g	Net Carbs: 8g
Protein: 3g	Total Fat: 12g	Calories: 159

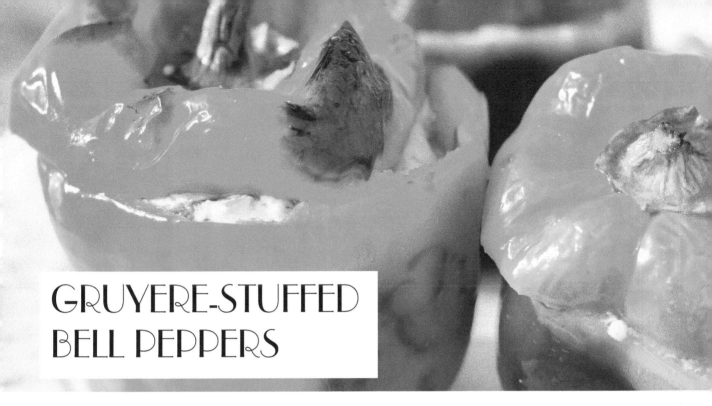

GRUYERE-STUFFED BELL PEPPERS

 10 minutes   **20 minutes**

INGREDIENTS

» 2 small bell peppers, any color
» 1 cup shredded Gruyere cheese
» 2 tablespoons fresh parsley, minced
» 1 clove garlic, peeled and minced
» 2 green onions, chopped
» 10 green olives, pitted and chopped

Essentials

» Salt and ground black pepper, to taste
» 2 tablespoons olive oil

Optional/ Garnish

» ¼ cup whole leaf basil

DIRECTIONS

1. Preheat oven to 375°F.

2. Cut off the tops of the bell peppers and remove the core and seeds. Rub the pepper with olive oil, place on a roasting pan, and roast for about 20 minutes. Allow to cool slightly.

3. In a small bowl combine the minced garlic, green onion, parsley, and olives. Add the shredded Gruyere and mix well.

4. Stuff each pepper with the cheese mixture.

5. Transfer back to the oven and cook for an additional 5 minutes.

6. Transfer to a serving plate, garnish with basil, and enjoy.

NUTRITION FACTS (PER SERVING)

Total Carbohydrates: 11g	Dietary Fiber: 3g	Net Carbs: 8g
Protein: 22g	Total Fat: 37g	Calories: 461

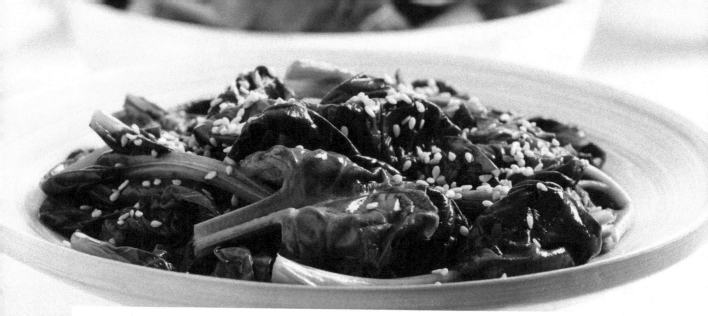

SESAME GARLIC SPINACH (GF)

 5 minutes   5 minutes   👥

INGREDIENTS

» 2 cups spinach, chopped
» 1 teaspoon toasted sesame seeds
» 2 garlic cloves, peeled and minced
» ½ tablespoon coconut aminos
» ½ teaspoon rice vinegar
» ½ teaspoon raw honey

Essentials

» 1 tablespoon peanut oil (use avocado oil for a paleo version)
» Ground black pepper, to taste

DIRECTIONS

1. Place the spinach in a large saucepan of boiling water and cook for 3-4 minutes until the greens wilt.

2. Transfer to a colander and rinse with cold water. Drain and squeeze with hands to remove as much water as possible. Place in a salad bowl.

3. To prepare the dressing: Combine the coconut aminos, peanut oil, rice vinegar, sesame seeds, garlic, honey, and pepper in a small bowl. Whisk until well combined.

4. Pour the dressing over the spinach and toss to coat.

5. Refrigerate for at least 1 hour before serving.

NUTRITION FACTS (PER SERVING)

Total Carbohydrates: 6g	Dietary Fiber: 1g	Net Carbs: 5g
Protein: 2g	Total Fat: 8g	Calories: 101

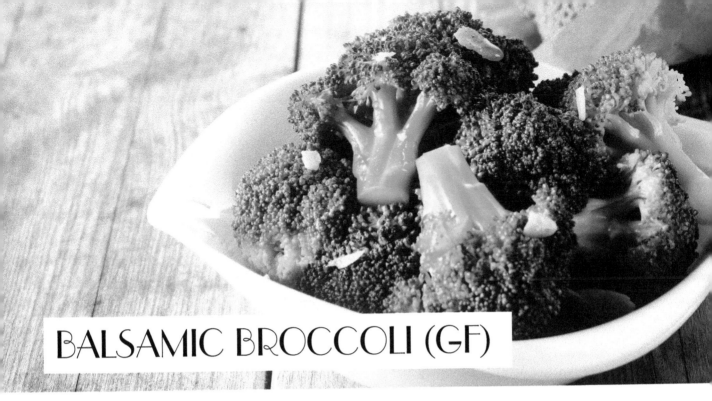

BALSAMIC BROCCOLI (GF)

 15 minutes   15 minutes   👤👤

INGREDIENTS

- » 1 large head of broccoli, cut into florets
- » 2 tablespoons balsamic vinegar
- » 2 garlic cloves, peeled and minced
- » ½ red onion, peeled and diced

Essentials

- » 2 tablespoons sesame oil
- » Salt and ground black pepper, to taste

DIRECTIONS

1. Preheat oven to 450°F.

2. In a large bowl, combine the broccoli with sesame oil. Season with salt and pepper to taste and mix well to coat.

3. Transfer the broccoli to a large baking dish lined with parchment and roast in the oven for 18-20 minutes until golden brown. Allow to cool and transfer to a salad bowl.

4. Whisk the balsamic vinegar, onion, and garlic together in a small bowl, season with salt and pepper, and pour over the roasted broccoli. Mix well to coat and enjoy.

NUTRITION FACTS (PER SERVING)

Total Carbohydrates: 8g	Dietary Fiber: 1g	Net Carbs: 7g
Protein: 1g	Total Fat: 14g	Calories: 159

DESSERTS/
SWEET SNACKS

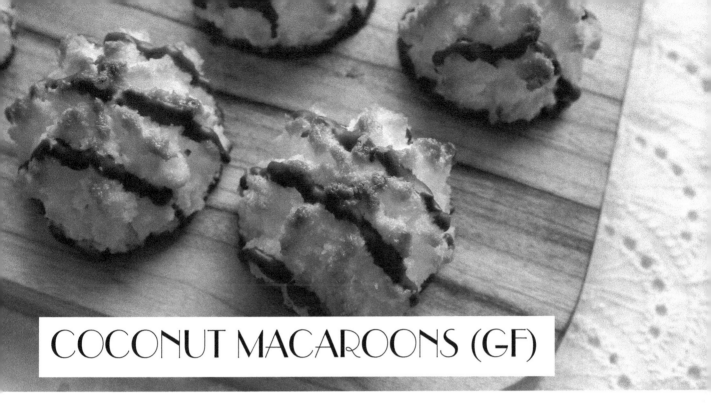

COCONUT MACAROONS (GF)

 10 minutes   **25 minutes**   **6 macaroons**

INGREDIENTS

» ½ cup shredded coconut
» ½ cup ground almonds
» 1 large egg white
» ¼ cup sugar substitute
» 1 ounce sugar-free chocolate chips (be sure these are gluten-free)
» 2 tablespoons butter

Essentials

» Salt, to taste

DIRECTIONS

1. Preheat the oven to 350°F.
2. Spread the shredded coconut and ground almonds evenly on a baking sheet lined with parchment paper.
3. Place in the oven and toast for 3-5 minutes until light golden and fragrant.
4. In a mixing bowl, beat the egg white with an electric mixer and gradually add sugar substitute. Once stiff peaks form, stir in the toasted coconut, almonds, and a pinch of salt.
5. Line a baking dish with parchment. Shape the mixture into small balls and arrange them on the prepared baking dish. You can shape them with your hands or use an ice cream scoop.
6. Bake in the oven for 15-18 minutes until their tops are golden brown.
7. In a small bowl, melt the butter and chocolate chips.
8. Once the macaroons are done, remove from the oven and let them cool for 5 minutes.
9. Drizzle the macaroons with chocolate and enjoy.

NUTRITION FACTS (PER SERVING)

Total Carbohydrates: 5g	**Dietary Fiber: 1g**	**Net Carbs: 4g**
Protein: 1g	**Total Fat: 8g**	**Calories: 102**

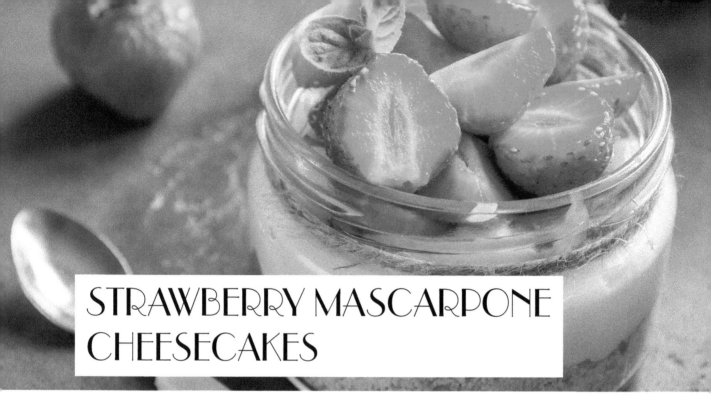

STRAWBERRY MASCARPONE CHEESECAKES

 10 minutes   0 minutes

INGREDIENTS

- » 4 ounces mascarpone
- » 7 strawberries
- » ¼ cup almond flour
- » ½ cup sugar substitute
- » ¼ cup crème fraiche
- » 1 teaspoon vanilla extract

Essentials

- » 3 tablespoons butter, melted

DIRECTIONS

1. To prepare the crust, combine the melted butter, almond flour, and about ⅔ of the sugar substitute in a bowl and mix well to combine.

2. Divide the mixture evenly into 2 serving bowls, lightly pressing with your hands.

3. To prepare the filling, puree the strawberries in a food processor, leaving 2 strawberries to the side for garnish.

4. Add the remaining sugar substitute, vanilla extract, mascarpone, and crème fraiche to the food processor. Blend until it reaches a smooth consistency.

5. Spoon the mixture over the crusts and allow it to chill in the refrigerator for at least 1 hour.

6. Slice the remaining strawberries and arrange on each bowl. Serve and enjoy.

NUTRITION FACTS (PER SERVING)

Total Carbohydrates: 8g	Dietary Fiber: 2g	Net Carbs: 6g
Protein: 17g	Total Fat: 31g	Calories: 442

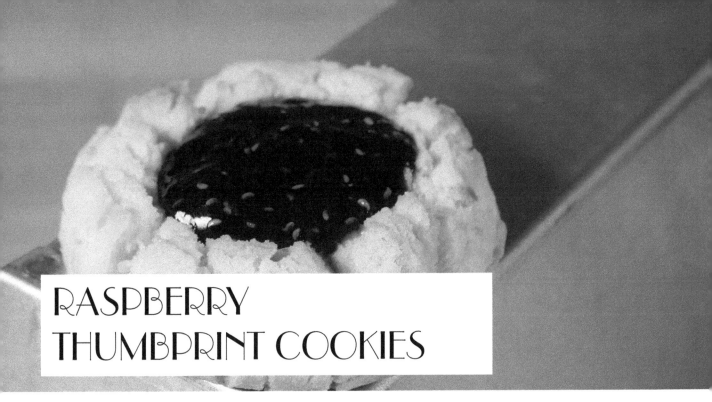

RASPBERRY THUMBPRINT COOKIES

 10 minutes   **12 minutes**   **10 cookies**

INGREDIENTS

- » 1 tablespoon coconut flour
- » 1 cup almond butter
- » 1 egg
- » ½ teaspoon vanilla extract
- » ⅔ cup sugar substitute
- » 3-4 tablespoons raspberry jam, no-sugar added

Essentials

- » ¼ teaspoon baking powder

DIRECTIONS

1. Preheat oven to 350°F.

2. Using an electric mixer, beat the egg together with the almond butter and sugar substitute. Add the coconut flour, baking powder, and vanilla extract. Mix well to form a smooth dough.

3. Shape the mixture into small balls and arrange on a baking sheet lined with parchment paper.

4. Make a slight indentation on the top each of the cookies with your thumb or the back of a spoon. Fill with about ½ teaspoon of the jam.

5. Bake in the oven for 10-12 minutes until the cookies are golden brown around the edges.

NUTRITION FACTS (PER SERVING)

Total Carbohydrates: 6g	Dietary Fiber: 3g	Net Carbs: 3g
Protein: 6g	Total Fat: 15g	Calories: 173

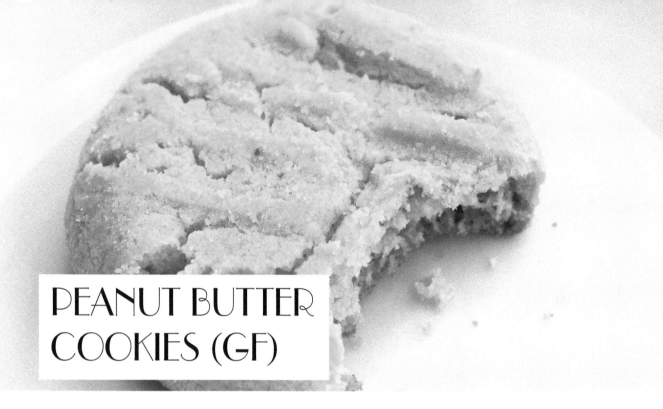

PEANUT BUTTER COOKIES (GF)

 10 minutes   🕐 **15 minutes**   👥 **12 cookies**

INGREDIENTS

» 1 cup peanut butter
» ½ cup almond flour
» ½ cup sugar substitute
» 2 eggs
» 1 teaspoon vanilla extract

Essentials

» ¼ teaspoon salt

DIRECTIONS

1. Preheat oven to 350°F.

2. Prepare a baking sheet with parchment paper or nonstick cooking spray.

3. Place the peanut butter, eggs, almond flour, sugar substitute, salt, and vanilla extract in a bowl and mix well with an electric mixer to form a smooth dough.

4. Shape the dough into walnut-size balls and arrange on the prepared baking sheet.

5. Using a fork, make crisscross marks on the cookies and bake in the oven for 16-18 minutes until golden brown.

NUTRITION FACTS (PER SERVING)

Total Carbohydrates: 6g	Dietary Fiber: 1g	Net Carbs: 4g
Protein: 4g	Total Fat: 5g	Calories: 96

62

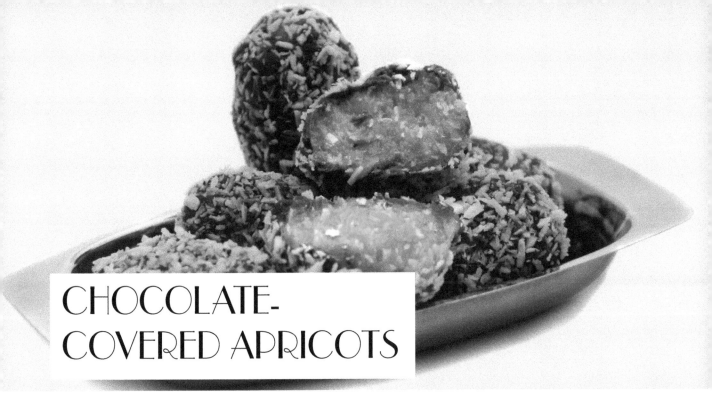

CHOCOLATE-COVERED APRICOTS

 15 minutes   15 minutes   18

INGREDIENTS

» ½ cup bittersweet chocolate chips
» 36 dried apricots
» ½ cup shredded coconut

DIRECTIONS

1. Place the chocolate chips in a microwave-safe bowl and microwave for 30 seconds. Stir the chocolate and continue microwaving in 30-second intervals until melted.

2. Coat half of each apricot with the melted chocolate and arrange on a baking sheet lined with parchment. Sprinkle the apricots with the shredded coconut.

3. Chill for at least 1 hour before serving.

NUTRITION FACTS (PER SERVING)

Total Carbohydrates: 4g	Dietary Fiber: 1g	Net Carbs: 3g
Protein: 0g	Total Fat: 1g	Calories: 349

BREAKFAST

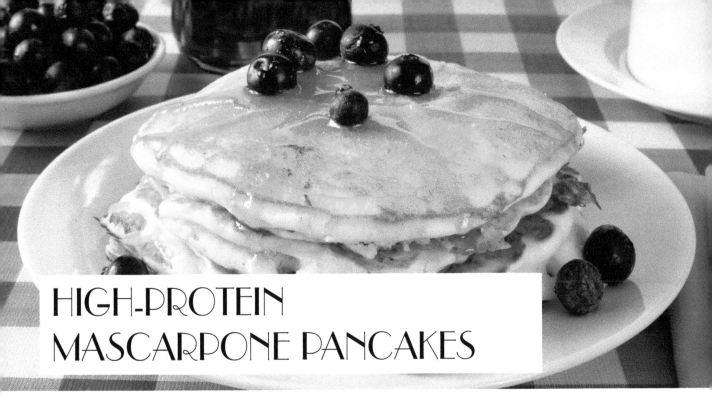

HIGH-PROTEIN MASCARPONE PANCAKES

 5 minutes   **10 minutes**

INGREDIENTS

- » 6 eggs
- » 1 cup mascarpone cheese
- » ¼ cup ground flaxseeds
- » ¼ cup chia seeds
- » 1 ½ teaspoons baking powder

Essentials

- » ½ teaspoon salt

Suggested Toppings

- Butter
- Low-carb syrup
- Sour cream
- Berries

DIRECTIONS

1. Combine the flaxseeds, chia seeds, baking powder, and salt in a bowl. Add the eggs to the dry ingredients one at a time, whisking well after each egg.
2. Add the mascarpone cheese and whisk until smooth. Alternatively, put all of the ingredients into a blender to achieve the same results. If you want to sweeten the batter, add about a teaspoon of sugar substitute at this point and mix well.
3. Spray a griddle or nonstick skillet with cooking oil spray and set over medium-high heat.
4. Use a large spoon or, preferably, a ladle (this is the perfect size for cooking pancakes) to pour the pancake batter into the skillet once the skillet is hot.
5. Allow the pancake to cook for about 2 minutes before carefully flipping it over with a spatula. Cook the other side for about 2 minutes. Adjust the timing accordingly if you would prefer your pancakes more or less browned.

NUTRITION FACTS (PER SERVING)

Total Carbohydrates: 12g	**Dietary Fiber: 4g**	**Net Carbs: 8g**
Protein: 33g	**Total Fat: 41g**	**Calories: 546**

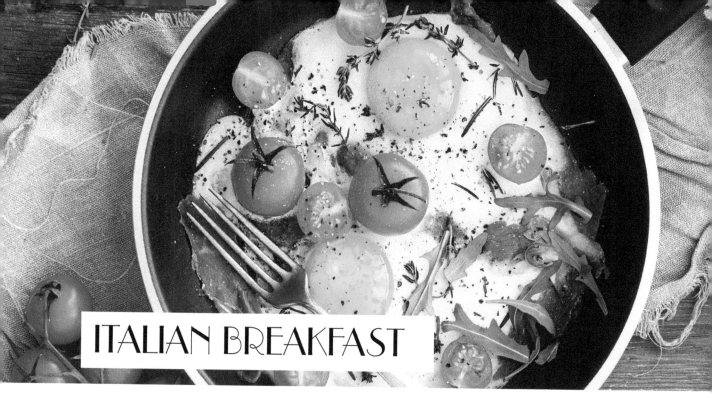

ITALIAN BREAKFAST

 15 minutes   10 minutes

INGREDIENTS

» 2 large eggs
» 3-4 slices prosciutto ham
» 1 clove garlic, peeled
» ½ cup arugula
» 10 cherry tomatoes, halved

Essentials

» Celtic sea salt
» Freshly ground black pepper
» 4 tablespoons butter

DIRECTIONS

1. Heat 1 tablespoon of butter in a small skillet over a medium-high heat.

2. Crack and fry the eggs, preferably sunny-side up, until the edges are golden (usually around 3-4 minutes). Remove from the pan and set to one side for the moment.

3. Next, crush the garlic clove. Add more butter, if needed, then add the garlic to the skillet and sauté until it begins to turn a golden brown. Add a dash of salt and pepper.

4. Sauté the halved tomatoes for about 2-3 minutes, turning halfway through.

NUTRITION FACTS (PER SERVING)

Total Carbohydrates: 5g	Dietary Fiber: 1g	Net Carbs: 4g
Protein: 7g	Total Fat: 17g	Calories: 189

66

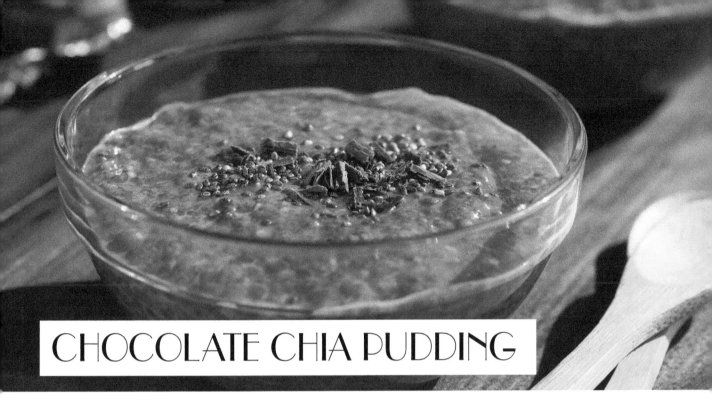

CHOCOLATE CHIA PUDDING

 2 minutes   3 minutes

INGREDIENTS

- » 2 tablespoons chia seeds
- » 4 scoops chocolate protein powder
- » 2 tablespoons ground flaxseeds
- » ½ cup almond flour
- » 1 cup canned coconut milk
- » 4 tablespoons hemp hearts

Essentials

- » ⅔ cup water
- » ¼ tablespoon ground cinnamon
- » ¼ tablespoon ground nutmeg

Suggested Toppings

- » Toasted almonds
- » Toasted coconut
- » Almond butter

DIRECTIONS

1. Combine the coconut milk and water together in a medium bowl. Combine the chia seeds, protein powder, flax seeds, almond flour, cinnamon, and nutmeg in a separate bowl.
2. Make a well in the dry ingredients and pour the milk/water mixture little by little into the dry ingredients while continuously mixing. Repeat until the ingredients are thoroughly mixed together. Cover the bowl and place in the refrigerator overnight. It is better to prepare this dish the night before serving to allow the flavors to combine and the seeds and flour to absorb the liquid.
3. The next day, place the mixture in a small saucepan and heat on low. Bring the mixture to a simmer and stir frequently until it thickens.
4. Stir in the hemp hearts just before serving.
5. Divide evenly between two bowls and add your favorite approved toppings.

NUTRITION FACTS (PER SERVING)

Total Carbohydrates: 20g	**Dietary Fiber: 10g**	**Net Carbs: 10g**
Protein: 38g	**Total Fat: 32g**	**Calories: 486**

CPSIA information can be obtained
at www.ICGtesting.com
Printed in the USA
BVHW091336110619
550700BV00019B/1297/P

9 780995 534506